Skeletal Muscle Health in Metabolic Diseases

Edited by

Hiroaki Eshima

Department of International Tourism
Sports Tourism Course
Nagasaki International University
Nagasaki, Japan

Ikuru Miura

Faculty of Sports and Health Science
Fukuoka University
Fukuoka, Japan

Yutaka Matsunaga

Faculty of Human Health
Kurume University
Kurume, Japan

&

Yuki Tomiga

Faculty of Sports and Health Science
Fukuoka University
Fukuoka, Japan

Skeletal Muscle Health in Metabolic Diseases

Editors: Hiroaki Eshima, Ikuru Miura, Yutaka Matsunaga & Yuki Tomiga

ISBN (Online): 978-981-5313-92-5

ISBN (Print): 978-981-5313-93-2

ISBN (Paperback): 978-981-5313-94-9

First published in 2024.

need for a court order if at any point you breach any terms of this License Agreement. In no event will any delay or failure by Bentham Science Publishers in enforcing your compliance with this License Agreement constitute a waiver of any of its rights.

3. You acknowledge that you have read this License Agreement, and agree to be bound by its terms and conditions. To the extent that any other terms and conditions presented on any website of Bentham Science Publishers conflict with, or are inconsistent with, the terms and conditions set out in this License Agreement, you acknowledge that the terms and conditions set out in this License Agreement shall prevail.

Bentham Science Publishers Pte. Ltd.
80 Robinson Road #02-00
Singapore 068898
Singapore
Email: subscriptions@benthamscience.net

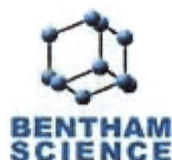

BENTHAM SCIENCE

CONTENTS

PREFACE

Metabolic diseases such as obesity and diabetes cause disruption of systemic energy metabolism and are major public health problems, affecting at least 2 billion people worldwide. The energy metabolism of the whole body is mainly regulated by skeletal muscle, liver, and brain. This book, entitled "Skeletal Muscle Health in Metabolic Disease", aims to clarify organ and tissue alterations in metabolic diseases, such as obesity, diabetes, and fatty liver.

The book comprises six chapters. The first chapter gives a background of metabolic diseases that affect cellular mechanisms in muscle cells and muscle tissue, especially glucose metabolism in skeletal muscle.

The skeletal muscle and liver share functions as metabolic organs, contributing to systemic metabolic regulation through mutual cooperation. The second chapter discusses the latest findings on the crosstalk between metabolic dysfunction-associated steatotic liver disease (MASLD) and skeletal muscles, which starts and progresses in association with obesity and its associated systemic metabolic abnormalities.

The third chapter focuses on nutrition, especially carbohydrate metabolism. Lipids are stored in the body mainly in the form of triglycerides, whereas carbohydrates are primarily stored in the liver and skeletal muscles in the form of glycogen. Glycogen utilization has also been shown to increase during exercise. When glycogen is depleted, exercise performance is impaired. Therefore, carbohydrate metabolism is important for exercise and the maintenance of organ and tissue homeostasis.

Metabolic diseases are closely associated with brain health and noncommunicable diseases, including type 2 diabetes. By contrast, exercise exerts its beneficial effects on the brain by releasing bioactive substances. The fourth chapter presents how metabolic diseases affect brain health and how exercise mitigates these detrimental effects, focusing particularly on the molecular mechanisms in the brain.

The subsequent five and six chapters discuss muscle atrophy and weakness and cellular mechanisms in metabolic disease. Muscle oxidative stress has been implicated in lipid species composition in the development of type 2 diabetes. Therefore, the sixth chapter discusses the impact of metabolic disorders, such as obesity and type 2 diabetes, on the regulation of lipid species and oxidative stress.

Hiroaki Eshima
Department of International Tourism
Sports Tourism Course
Nagasaki International University
Nagasaki, Japan

Ikuru Miura
Faculty of Sports and Health Science
Fukuoka University
Fukuoka, Japan

Yutaka Matsunaga
Faculty of Human Health
Kurume University
Kurume, Japan

&

Yuki Tomiga
Faculty of Sports and Health Science
Fukuoka University
Fukuoka, Japan

List of Contributors

Hiroaki Eshima   Department of International Tourism, Sports Tourism Course, Nagasaki International University, Nagasaki, Japan

Ikuru Miura   Faculty of Sports and Health Science, Fukuoka University, Fukuoka, Japan

Yutaka Matsunaga   Faculty of Human Health, Kurume University, Kurume, Japan

Yuki Tomiga   Faculty of Sports and Health Science, Fukuoka University, Fukuoka, Japan

CHAPTER 1

Muscle Glucose Metabolism in Metabolic Diseases

Hiroaki Eshima[1,*]

[1] *Department of International Tourism, Sports Tourism Course, Nagasaki International University, Nagasaki, Japan*

Abstract: Metabolic diseases such as obesity and diabetes cause disruption of systemic energy metabolism and are major public health problems, with at least 2 billion people affected worldwide. Skeletal muscle tissue makes a substantial contribution to promoting energy efficiency because it remodels cellular size, composition, and function in response to various nutritional changes. However, metabolic diseases such as impaired insulin sensitivity can dynamically affect the metabolism of skeletal muscle. A deeper understanding of myopathology in metabolic disorders may provide clues for therapeutic strategies to promote skeletal muscle health and improve the overall quality of life. This chapter presents how metabolic diseases *via* cellular mechanisms affect muscle cells and muscle tissue, especially glucose metabolism in skeletal muscle.

Keywords: Diabetes, Glucose, Obesity, Metabolism, Skeletal muscle.

INTRODUCTION

Diabetes and obesity have a high risk of leading to diseases, including myocardial infarction and stroke, which affect life expectancy, and thus therapeutic strategies are needed [1]. A major feature of metabolic disease is insulin resistance. Insulin resistance is associated with obesity and type 2 diabetes mellitus (T2DM). It is generally defined as a reduction in the ability of the body to absorb blood glucose from circulation in response to insulin. Glucose is the main nutrition for energy consumption, but excess blood glucose is an index for obesity and T2DM. Insulin resistance from skeletal muscle is commonly viewed as the critical component of whole-body insulin resistance because the muscle is the most important tissue for insulin-stimulated glucose disposal [2].

Carbohydrates, lipids, and proteins all ultimately break down into glucose and then serve as the primary metabolic fuel in a mammalian cell. Glycogen in skel-

* **Corresponding author Hiroaki Eshima:** Department of International Tourism, Sports Tourism Course, Nagasaki International University, Nagasaki, Japan; E-mail: heshima@niu.ac.jp

etal muscles contains approximately as much as 50,000 glucose moeties. However, the large increase in muscle glycogen is generally associated with insulin resistance in the glucose transport process [3, 4]. Insulin activates the glycogen synthase pathway, whereas glycogen synthesis in muscle is markedly reduced in T2DM [5, 6]. Despite many years of research, the molecular mechanisms by which metabolic disease promotes insulin resistance in skeletal muscle are not fully understood.

Recent research focused on how lipid species affect glucose metabolism in skeletal muscles. Lipids were also used as molecules to probe the basic mechanisms of ion fragmentation following electron ionization [7]. However, fundamental studies using mass spectrometry analysis of lipids demonstrate that lipid species are associated with insulin resistance in obesity and diabetes [8 - 11]. This chapter presents the cellular and molecular mechanisms of obesity- and diabetes-induced insulin resistance in skeletal muscle.

MUSCLE GLUCOSE TRANSPORTER IN OBESITY AND DIABETES

Glucose is a key metabolic substrate for the whole body. Muscle tissues require glucose as an energy source for adenosine triphosphate (ATP) production [12]. Glucose metabolism starts with transport across the plasma membrane [13]. Skeletal muscles take up glucose in response to insulin stimulation and exercise. The insulin receptor (IR), insulin receptor substrates (IRS), and phosphatidylinositol 3-kinase (PI3K) activation are essential components of the insulin-induced response. Eventually, blood glucose is taken into intramyocellular through glucose transporter 4 (GLUT4) translocation [14, 15]. GLUT4 is an insulin-regulated glucose transporter that is responsible for glucose uptake in muscle. It is mainly located in intracellular vesicles in the absence of insulin [16]. Obesity and T2DM are strongly linked to the development of insulin resistance within the skeletal muscles [17]. In 1975, Kemmer *et al.* demonstrated that the skeletal muscles of obese rats are insulin-resistant with respect to both glucose-transport mechanisms and intracellular pathways of glucose metabolism [18]. Consistent with this, the expression of GLUT4 can explain the insulin-resistant glucose uptake characteristic of dietary-induced obesity [19]. A previous study revealed that transgenic overexpression of GLUT4 enhances glucose tolerance in lean and obese mice [20]. Taken together, increasing muscle GLUT4 content is an important target for improving glucose tolerance in obesity.

The main molecule pathway for glucose uptake through GLUT4 is the PI3K/AKT signaling pathway. The PI3K/AKT pathway is a central regulator in cellular physiology for growth factor signals and critical cellular processes [21]. PI3K and serine/threonine kinase 1 (Akt) signaling is important for insulin-stimulated glucose uptake in skeletal muscle tissues. AKT phosphorylates are involved in the regulation of GLUT4 translocation [22]. PI3K/AKT signaling pathway exists in various organs, but obesity and T2DM impair PI3K/AKT signaling [22]. Sano *et al*. demonstrated that insulin increases the phosphorylation of AS160 and GLUT4 translocation in 3T3-L1 adipocytes [23]. In human skeletal muscles, exercise increases AS160 phosphorylation without insulin infusion [24]. Similarly, obese rodent muscles decrease glucose uptake with decreased AS160 phosphorylation on Ser588 with or without insulin stimulation [25].

AMP-activated protein kinase (AMPK) increases glucose uptake through PI3K/Akt signaling. For instance, loss of skeletal muscle AMPK exacerbates glucose intolerance and insulin resistance in obese people, resulting in a significant decrease in glucose uptake in skeletal muscles [26]. Indeed, loss of AMPK activity has been observed in the skeletal muscle of patients with obesity and diabetes [27, 28]. 5-Aminoimidazole-4-carboxamide ribonucleoside (AICAR) reportedly activates AMPK and stimulates glucose uptake by skeletal muscle [29], suggesting a drug target to facilitate muscle glucose uptake in obesity and diabetes [30]. Long-term AICAR improves glucose metabolism in insulin-resistant obese mice, which can be explained by effects on muscle glucose uptake [31]. However, a previous report has reported that the stimulatory effects of AICAR on glucose uptake are reduced in older men, irrespective of type 2 diabetes, suggesting that AICAR has only a limited therapeutic effect on older type 2 diabetic skeletal muscles [32].

TBC1D1 and TBC1D4, the two Rab GTPase-activating proteins, are closely related to the GLUT4 translocation to the plasma membrane, resulting in increased glucose uptake [33]. The phosphorylation of TBC1D1 and TBC1D4 has been defined as targets for the AKT and the AMPK [34]. Insulin increases in AS160 phosphorylation in skeletal muscle tissues [35] and cells [36]. Deletion of phosphorylated AS160 exhibits reduced insulin-induced GLUT4 translocation in adipocytes and muscle cells [23, 37]. Therefore, AS160 phosphorylation induces glucose uptake into muscles through the translocation of GLUT4 vesicles. On the other hand, insulin-stimulated AS160 phosphorylation is reduced in T2DM [38]. However, reduced muscle glucose uptake of obesity is not associated with the AKT/AS160 content [39]. Therefore, underlying mechanisms for the impaired glucose uptake in metabolic disease are not completely understood.

In type 1 diabetic rodent models induced streptozocin, NPC43 can effectively increase glucose uptake by activating PI3K, Akt, and AS160 pathways through insulin receptors [40]. Akt and AMPK phosphorylated proteins to vesicle traffic appear to be dependent on linking to small GTPase of the Rab family [41]. When activated, Akt by insulin or muscle contraction phosphorylates AS160 and

TBC1D1. Muscle contraction through both energy depletion and increased intracellular calcium leads to activation of AMPK *via* LKB1 and Ca^{2+}/calmodulin-dependent protein kinase kinase (CaMKK). These proteins lead to AS160 and TBC1D1 phosphorylation. This is thought to regulate the function of these proteins and GLUT4 trafficking by largely uncharacterized mechanisms independent of insulin receptor substrate. On the other hand, overexpression of TBC1D1 does not alter glucose uptake-induced insulin or contraction [42].

MUSCLE GLUCOSE TRANSPORTER IN EXERCISE

Physical exercise is an effective preventive method to prevent obesity and T2DM [43, 44]. It is well established that exercise improves glucose metabolism with T2DM, and adaptations to skeletal muscles are essential for this improvement [17]. Glucose uptake into muscle increases depending on exercise intensity and exercise duration in healthy humans [45]. Exercise increases muscle glucose uptake in diabetic patients like healthy people [46]. The most famous feature of exercise is insulin-independent glucose uptake. Genetic rodent models of muscle-specific insulin receptor knockout do not increase exercise-induced glucose uptake [47], suggesting that exercise promotes insulin-independent signaling pathways for increased glucose uptake. Exercise changes energy status, resulting in increased AMP levels and then induced activation of AMPK. These are the most widely studied proteins implicated in glucose uptake in response to exercise [48]. Meanwhile, AS160, a Rab GTPase-activating protein, is involved in AMPK signaling to glucose uptake. For instance, AICAR increases both AMPK and phosphorylation of AS160 by insulin-independent mechanisms [49]. CaMKII, AS160, and TBC1D1 are also linked to a mechanism for AMPK signaling [50] (Fig. **1**).

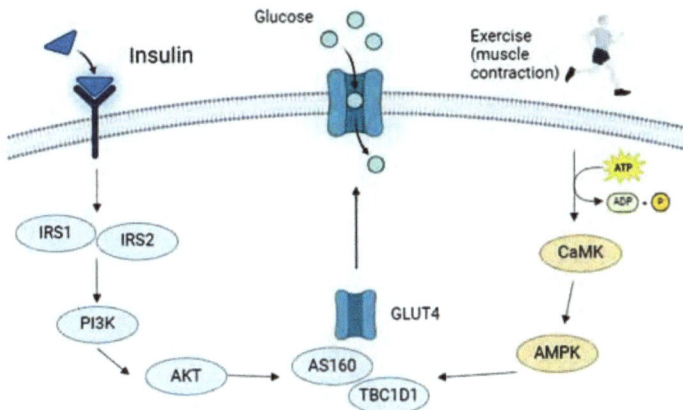

Fig. (1). Schematic diagram of the cellular mechanisms for glucose uptake induced by insulin- and muscle contraction (Exercise).

Exercise training is also an important recommendation for the management of diabetes due to improving insulin sensitivity in patients [51]. The review from Jensen *et al.* discusses the following: 1. the insulin sensitivity is increased for up to a single bout of exercise [52]. 2. Exercise training improves insulin sensitivity and glucose uptake [53]. Therefore, exercise can improve dysfunctional insulin pathways and augment glucose uptake in insulin resistance to normalize glycemic control in metabolic disease [54]. On the other hand, some training protocols fail to improve glucose tolerance and prevent a decrease in body weight and mass of adipose tissue [55]. Exercise training decreases glucose uptake during exercise despite a large increase in GLUT4 protein content [45]. For instance, eccentric exercise impairs glucose uptake in skeletal muscle [56]. Indeed, muscle GLUT-4 content is decreased after eccentric contractions [57]. Another study demonstrates that metabolic pathway dysregulations in obesity were improved with vigorous physical exercise [58]. In addition, another study demonstrated that mechanical overload stimulates muscle glucose uptake independent of GLUT4 content [59]. A previous study using the genetic rodent models (muscle-specific GLUT4 knockout) confirmed that GLUT4 is not necessary for overload-induced muscle glucose uptake [61]. GLUT1 also does not mediate basal muscle glucose uptake induced by overload, suggesting that different exercise protocols (eccentric contraction, mechanical overload, endurance running, *etc.*) have different mechanisms for muscle glucose transporter [62] (Fig. **2**).

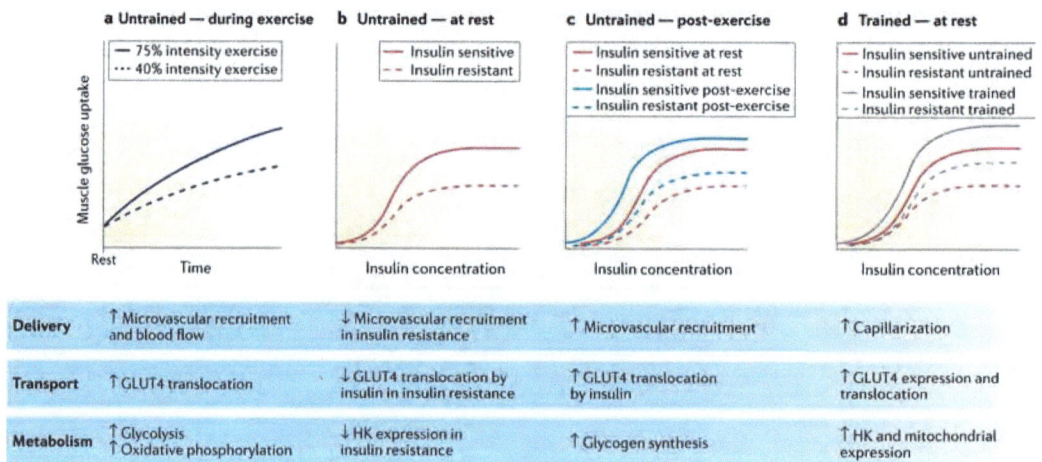

Fig. (2). The influence of exercise (acute and or training) on insulin action. These are summarized in Jensen *et al.* [60].

Obese and type 2 diabetic subjects have attenuated AMPK and phosphorylation of AS160 induced by exercise [28]. GLUT4 translocation is impaired in T2DM, whereas exercise results in a normal increase in GLUT4 translocation and glucose uptake. Genetic loss of AMPK function in skeletal muscle has been identified as decreased glucose uptake, but it is unclear in basal systemic glucose metabolism [63]. A recent study demonstrated that a non-selective activator of all AMPK complexes activator caused a decrease in blood glucose in diabetic mice [64]. In contrast, metformin, an activator on AMPK, did not affect glucose uptake at relevant pharmacological concentrations in initial reports [65]. These phenomena indicate that exercise-induced glucose uptake in diabetic patients could not be explained by action of AMPK activation.

MUSCLE LIPID AND INSULIN RESISTANCE IN OBESITY AND DIABETES

The accumulation of intramyocellular lipids may lead to insulin resistance in skeletal muscle. Lipid intermediates directly impair muscle insulin signaling. *De novo* lipid synthesis might contribute to glucose disposal when glycogen stores are filled. Muscle insulin resistance caused by lipid accumulation alters the subcellular localization of diacylglycerols (DAGs) and ceramides, accelerates peripheral inflammation and damage, and leads to heart failure, nonalcoholic fatty liver disease, obesity, renal anemia, and sarcopenia besides diabetes [66]. Recent research focused on how ceramides and phospholipids alter muscle composition and cause insulin resistance during obesity and diabetes. Ceramides induce insulin resistance in cultured cells by inhibitory effects on insulin signaling [67]. In obesity, the reduction of insulin stimulates glucose uptake and is associated with increased intramyocellular ceramide content [68]. Importantly, sarcopenia involves ceramide content, but insulin resistance was not fully investigated [69]. Previous studies demonstrate that sphingolipid mediators, including ceramide and sphingosine 1-phosphate, influence obesity and glucose metabolism [70 - 72]. Cellular accumulation of ceramide causes cell death, including pancreatic β-cell survival, and then deteriorates insulin resistance in the liver and the skeletal muscle. The sphingosine 1-phosphate activator improves obesity and associated metabolic disorders, whereas that of another type of phosphate has the opposite effect. The sphingosine kinase may affect glucose uptake [73]. However, a recent study suggests that altered phospholipid composition may affect glucose uptake/insulin action in skeletal muscle [74].

Phospholipids are a class of lipids and have a hydrophilic "head" containing a phosphate group and two hydrophobic "tails" derived from fatty acids. Previous studies identified ceramides and phosphatidylcholines (PC, the main molecular species of phospholipid) as promising biomarkers for cardiovascular disease [75 - 78]. Skeletal muscle consists of ~60% PC, ~30% phosphatidylethanolamine (PE), ~10% cardiolipin (CL), ~5% phosphatidylinositol (PI), phosphatidylserine (PS), lyso-PC, and sphingomyelin [79]. Muscle phospholipid and insulin resistance with obesity are well investigated [9, 11, 80, 81]. The phosphatidylethanolamine (PE) methyltransferase regulates obesity and insulin-stimulated glucose uptake in skeletal muscle in mice [82]. Consistent with this, lysophospholipids are associated with muscle insulin sensitivity in obesity in humans and mice [74] (Figs. **3** and **4**). These findings suggest that the alteration of phospholipid composition influences glucose uptake into muscle.

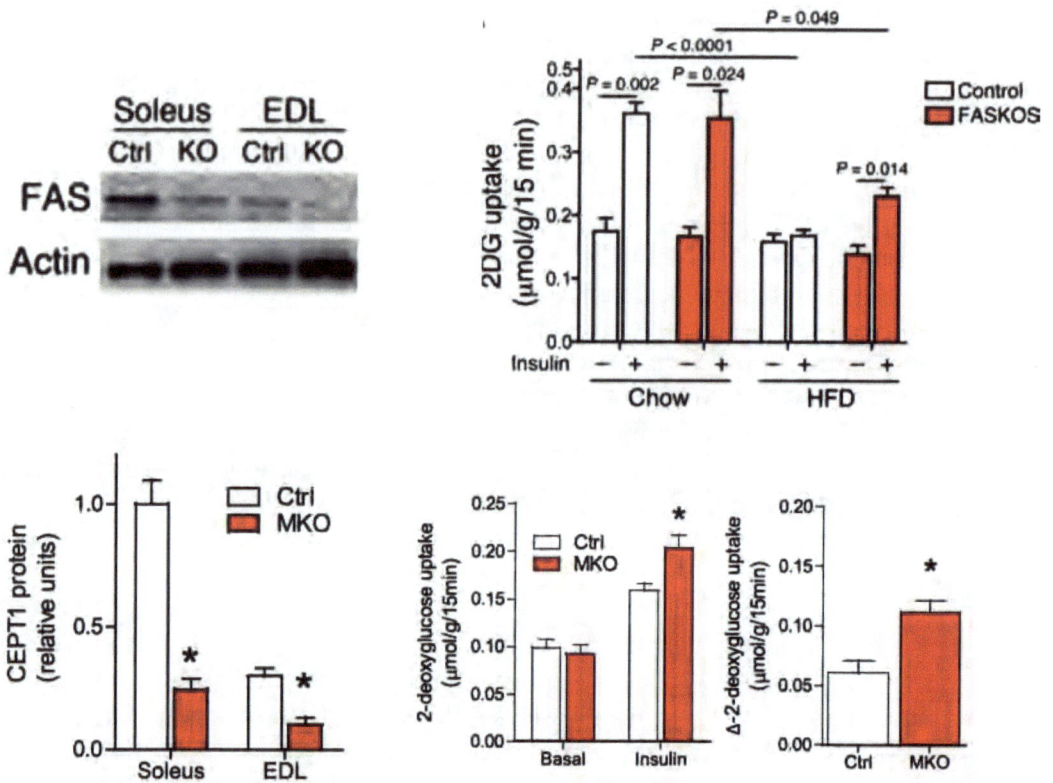

Fig. (3). The fatty acid synthase (FAS) was increased in insulin resistance. Skeletal muscle-specific knockout of FAS (FASKOS) protected mice from insulin resistance and glucose uptake. In the choline/ethanolamine phosphotransferase 1 (CEPT1), the terminal enzyme in the Kennedy pathway of phospholipid synthesis, skeletal muscle-specific knockout mice (MKO) increase muscle insulin sensitivity. From [9, 11].

Sarcolipin is a transmembrane protein that catalyzes the ATP-dependent transport of Ca^{2+} from the cytosol into the SR lumen and regulates Ca-ATPase activity in skeletal muscle. It is also involved in the regulation of mitochondrial biogenesis and oxidative metabolism in muscle [83]. Ablation of sarcolipin impairs the maintenance of core body temperature from cold exposure and causes hypothermia, excessive obesity, and glucose intolerance [84]. Conversely, overexpression of sarcolipin increased muscle-based thermogenesis through SERCA activity [85]. These studies suggest that the heat release rate by the sarcolipin and SERCA are associated with fat/glucose metabolism and basal metabolic rate. A previous study has suggested that sarcolipin may incorporate into phospholipid bilayers [86], but the influence of sarcolipin on phospholipids has not been completely explored.

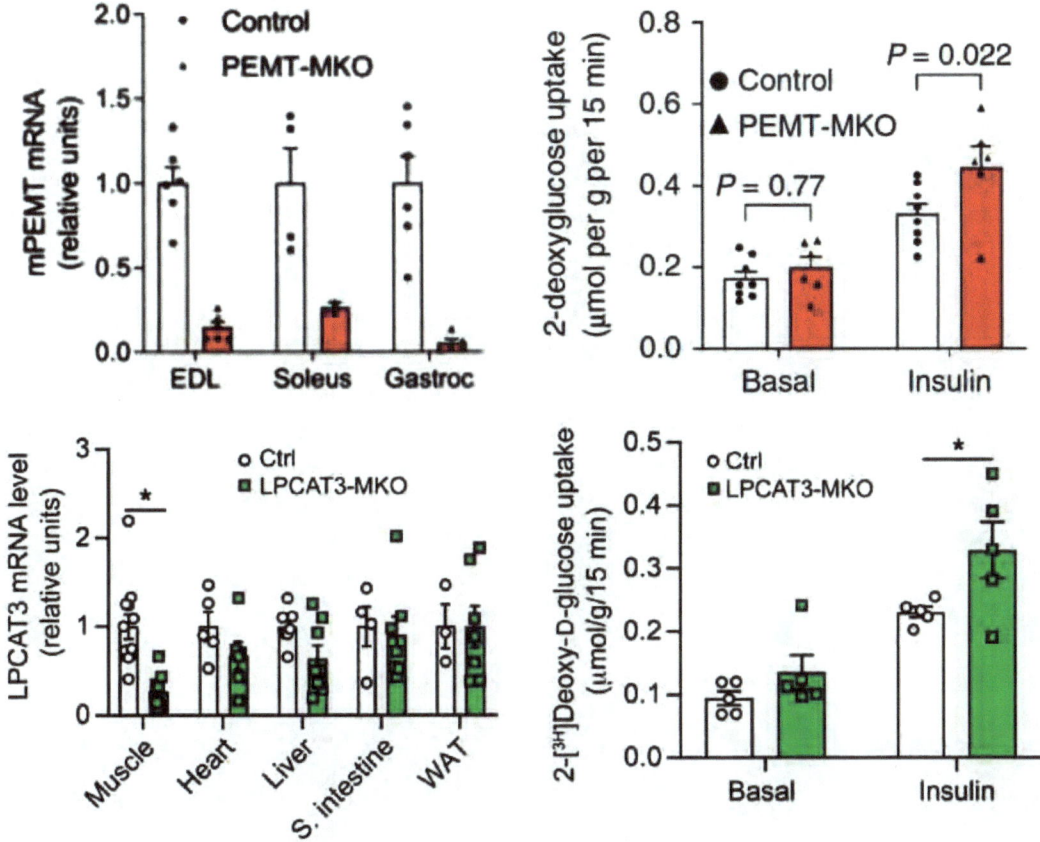

Fig. (4). In phosphatidylethanolamine methyltransferase (PEMT) and the lysophosphatidylcholine acyltransferase 3 (LPCAT3), skeletal muscle-specific knockout mice (MKO) increase muscle insulin sensitivity. From [74, 82].

Taken together, these findings might show that manipulation of lipid composition could promote protection from obesity and diabetes due to improved skeletal muscle energy supply (Fig. **5**).

CONCLUDING REMARKS

This chapter explained glucose metabolism, especially glucose uptake in skeletal muscles in obesity and type 2 diabetes. Many studies demonstrate the underlying mechanism of insulin- and contraction-induced glucose uptake, but the potential mechanism in metabolic disorders has not been fully clarified. In particular, the accumulation of lipids contributes to metabolic disorders, so lipid species such as ceramide, phospholipid, and DAG may regulate muscle glucose metabolism.

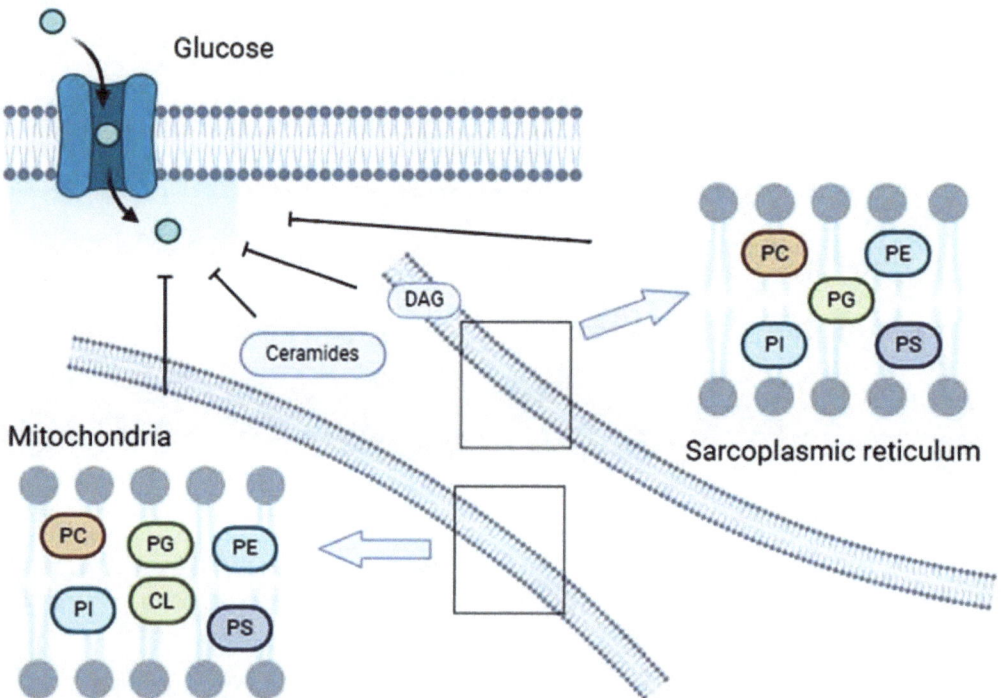

Fig. (5). Schematic diagram of the cellular lipid species for glucose uptake.

REFERENCES

[1] Ma CX, Ma XN, Guan CH, Li YD, Mauricio D, Fu SB. Cardiovascular disease in type 2 diabetes mellitus: progress toward personalized management. Cardiovasc Diabetol 2022; 21(1): 74.
[http://dx.doi.org/10.1186/s12933-022-01516-6] [PMID: 35568946]

[2] Turcotte LP, Fisher JS. Skeletal muscle insulin resistance: roles of fatty acid metabolism and exercise. Phys Ther 2008; 88(11): 1279-96.
[http://dx.doi.org/10.2522/ptj.20080018] [PMID: 18801860]

[3] Richter EA, Hansen SA, Hansen BF. Mechanisms limiting glycogen storage in muscle during prolonged insulin stimulation. Am J Physiol 1988; 255(5 Pt 1): E621-8.
[PMID: 3142271]

[4] Kawanaka K, Nolte LA, Han DH, Hansen PA, Holloszy JO. Mechanisms underlying impaired GLUT-

4 translocation in glycogen-supercompensated muscles of exercised rats. Am J Physiol Endocrinol Metab 2000; 279(6): E1311-8.
[http://dx.doi.org/10.1152/ajpendo.2000.279.6.E1311] [PMID: 11093919]

[5]   Jensen J, Rustad PI, Kolnes AJ, Lai YC. The role of skeletal muscle glycogen breakdown for regulation of insulin sensitivity by exercise. Front Physiol 2011; 2: 112.
[http://dx.doi.org/10.3389/fphys.2011.00112] [PMID: 22232606]

[6]   Shulman GI, Rothman DL, Jue T, Stein P, DeFronzo RA, Shulman RG. Quantitation of muscle glycogen synthesis in normal subjects and subjects with non-insulin-dependent diabetes by 13C nuclear magnetic resonance spectroscopy. N Engl J Med 1990; 322(4): 223-8.
[http://dx.doi.org/10.1056/NEJM199001253220403] [PMID: 2403659]

[7]   Vanlear GE, Mclafferty FW. Biochemical aspects of high-resolution mass spectrometry. Annu Rev Biochem 1969; 38(1): 289-322.
[http://dx.doi.org/10.1146/annurev.bi.38.070169.001445] [PMID: 4896241]

[8]   Jensen-Urstad APL, Song H, Lodhi IJ, *et al.* Nutrient-dependent phosphorylation channels lipid synthesis to regulate PPARα. J Lipid Res 2013; 54(7): 1848-59.
[http://dx.doi.org/10.1194/jlr.M036103] [PMID: 23585690]

[9]   Funai K, Song H, Yin L, *et al.* Muscle lipogenesis balances insulin sensitivity and strength through calcium signaling. J Clin Invest 2013; 123(3): 1229-40.
[http://dx.doi.org/10.1172/JCI65726] [PMID: 23376793]

[10]   Lodhi IJ, Yin L, Jensen-Urstad APL, *et al.* Inhibiting adipose tissue lipogenesis reprograms thermogenesis and PPARγ activation to decrease diet-induced obesity. Cell Metab 2012; 16(2): 189-201.
http://dx.doi.org/10.1016/j.cmet.2012.06.013] [PMID: 22863804]

[11]   Funai K, Lodhi IJ, Spears LD, *et al.* Skeletal muscle phospholipid metabolism regulates insulin sensitivity and contractile function. Diabetes 2016; 65(2): 358-70.
[http://dx.doi.org/10.2337/db15-0659] [PMID: 26512026]

[12]   Devaskar SU, Mueckler MM. The mammalian glucose transporters. Pediatr Res 1992; 31(1): 1-13.
[http://dx.doi.org/10.1203/00006450-199201000-00001] [PMID: 1594323]

[13]   Wheeler TJ, Hinkle PC. The glucose transporter of mammalian cells. Annu Rev Physiol 1985; 47(1): 503-17.
[http://dx.doi.org/10.1146/annurev.ph.47.030185.002443] [PMID: 3888079]

[14]   Czech MP. PIP2 and PIP3: complex roles at the cell surface. Cell 2000; 100(6): 603-6.
[http://dx.doi.org/10.1016/S0092-8674(00)80696-0] [PMID: 10761925]

[15]   Heller-Harrison RA, Morin M, Guilherme A, Czech MP. Insulin-mediated targeting of phosphatidylinositol 3-kinase to GLUT4-containing vesicles. J Biol Chem 1996; 271(17): 10200-4.
[http://dx.doi.org/10.1074/jbc.271.17.10200] [PMID: 8626583]

[16]   Donkerlo TW. [Cholesterol determination and age]. Ned Tijdschr Geneeskd 1990; 134(45): 2203-4. [Cholesterol determination and age].
[PMID: 2247191]

[17]   DeFronzo RA, Tripathy D. Skeletal muscle insulin resistance is the primary defect in type 2 diabetes. Diabetes Care 2009; 32(Suppl 2) (Suppl. 2): S157-63.
[http://dx.doi.org/10.2337/dc09-S302] [PMID: 19875544]

[18]   Kemmer FW, Berger M, Herberg L, Gries FA, Wirdeier A, Becker K. Glucose metabolism in perfused skeletal muscle. Demonstration of insulin resistance in the obese Zucker rat. Biochem J 1979; 178(3): 733-41.
[http://dx.doi.org/10.1042/bj1780733] [PMID: 454379]

[19]   Kahn BB, Pedersen O. Suppression of GLUT4 expression in skeletal muscle of rats that are obese from high fat feeding but not from high carbohydrate feeding or genetic obesity. Endocrinology 1993;

132(1): 13-22.
[http://dx.doi.org/10.1210/endo.132.1.8419118] [PMID: 8419118]

[20] Atkinson BJ, Griesel BA, King CD, Josey MA, Olson AL. Moderate GLUT4 overexpression improves insulin sensitivity and fasting triglyceridemia in high-fat diet-fed transgenic mice. Diabetes 2013; 62(7): 2249-58.
[http://dx.doi.org/10.2337/db12-1146] [PMID: 23474483]

[21] Abeyrathna P, Su Y. The critical role of Akt in cardiovascular function. Vascul Pharmacol 2015; 74: 38-48.
[http://dx.doi.org/10.1016/j.vph.2015.05.008] [PMID: 26025205]

[22] Huang X, Liu G, Guo J, Su Z. The PI3K/AKT pathway in obesity and type 2 diabetes. Int J Biol Sci 2018; 14(11): 1483-96.
[http://dx.doi.org/10.7150/ijbs.27173] [PMID: 30263000]

[23] Sano H, Kane S, Sano E, *et al.* Insulin-stimulated phosphorylation of a Rab GTPase-activating protein regulates GLUT4 translocation. J Biol Chem 2003; 278(17): 14599-602.
[http://dx.doi.org/10.1074/jbc.C300063200] [PMID: 12637568]

[24] Pehmøller C, Brandt N, Birk JB, *et al.* Exercise alleviates lipid-induced insulin resistance in human skeletal muscle-signaling interaction at the level of TBC1 domain family member 4. Diabetes 2012; 61(11): 2743-52.
[http://dx.doi.org/10.2337/db11-1572] [PMID: 22851577]

[25] Castorena CM, Arias EB, Sharma N, Cartee GD. Postexercise improvement in insulin-stimulated glucose uptake occurs concomitant with greater AS160 phosphorylation in muscle from normal and insulin-resistant rats. Diabetes 2014; 63(7): 2297-308.
[http://dx.doi.org/10.2337/db13-1686] [PMID: 24608437]

[26] Fujii N, Ho RC, Manabe Y, *et al.* Ablation of AMP-activated protein kinase alpha2 activity exacerbates insulin resistance induced by high-fat feeding of mice. Diabetes 2008; 57(11): 2958-66.
[http://dx.doi.org/10.2337/db07-1187] [PMID: 18728234]

[27] Bandyopadhyay GK, Yu JG, Ofrecio J, Olefsky JM. Increased malonyl-CoA levels in muscle from obese and type 2 diabetic subjects lead to decreased fatty acid oxidation and increased lipogenesis; thiazolidinedione treatment reverses these defects. Diabetes 2006; 55(8): 2277-85.
[http://dx.doi.org/10.2337/db06-0062] [PMID: 16873691]

[28] Sriwijitkamol A, Coletta DK, Wajcberg E, *et al.* Effect of acute exercise on AMPK signaling in skeletal muscle of subjects with type 2 diabetes: a time-course and dose-response study. Diabetes 2007; 56(3): 836-48.
[http://dx.doi.org/10.2337/db06-1119] [PMID: 17327455]

[29] Sakoda H, Ogihara T, Anai M, *et al.* Activation of AMPK is essential for AICAR-induced glucose uptake by skeletal muscle but not adipocytes. Am J Physiol Endocrinol Metab 2002; 282(6): E1239-44.
[http://dx.doi.org/10.1152/ajpendo.00455.2001] [PMID: 12006353]

[30] McIntyre EA, Halse R, Yeaman SJ, Walker M. Cultured muscle cells from insulin-resistant type 2 diabetes patients have impaired insulin, but normal 5-amino-4-imidazolecarboxamide riboside-stimulated, glucose uptake. J Clin Endocrinol Metab 2004; 89(7): 3440-8.
[http://dx.doi.org/10.1210/jc.2003-031919] [PMID: 15240629]

[31] Song XM, Fiedler M, Galuska D, *et al.* 5-Aminoimidazole-4-carboxamide ribonucleoside treatment improves glucose homeostasis in insulin-resistant diabetic (ob/ob) mice. Diabetologia 2002; 45(1): 56-65.
[http://dx.doi.org/10.1007/s125-002-8245-8] [PMID: 11845224]

[32] Babraj JA, Mustard K, Sutherland C, *et al.* Blunting of AICAR-induced human skeletal muscle glucose uptake in type 2 diabetes is dependent on age rather than diabetic status. Am J Physiol Endocrinol Metab 2009; 296(5): E1042-8.

[http://dx.doi.org/10.1152/ajpendo.90811.2008] [PMID: 19190259]

[33]   Peifer-Weiß L, Al-Hasani H, Chadt A. AMPK and beyond: the signaling network controlling rabgaps and contraction-mediated glucose uptake in skeletal muscle. Int J Mol Sci 2024; 25(3): 1910.
[http://dx.doi.org/10.3390/ijms25031910] [PMID: 38339185]

[34]   Espelage L, Al-Hasani H, Chadt A. RabGAPs in skeletal muscle function and exercise. J Mol Endocrinol 2020; 64(1): R1-R19.
[http://dx.doi.org/10.1530/JME-19-0143] [PMID: 31627187]

[35]   Cartee GD, Wojtaszewski JFP. Role of Akt substrate of 160 kDa in insulin-stimulated and contraction-stimulated glucose transport. Appl Physiol Nutr Metab 2007; 32(3): 557-66.
[http://dx.doi.org/10.1139/H07-026] [PMID: 17510697]

[36]   Kane S, Sano H, Liu SCH, *et al.* A method to identify serine kinase substrates. Akt phosphorylates a novel adipocyte protein with a Rab GTPase-activating protein (GAP) domain. J Biol Chem 2002; 277(25): 22115-8.
[http://dx.doi.org/10.1074/jbc.C200198200] [PMID: 11994271]

[37]   Thong FSL, Dugani CB, Klip A. Turning signals on and off: GLUT4 traffic in the insulin-signaling highway. Physiology (Bethesda) 2005; 20(4): 271-84.
[http://dx.doi.org/10.1152/physiol.00017.2005] [PMID: 16024515]

[38]   Karlsson HKR, Zierath JR, Kane S, Krook A, Lienhard GE, Wallberg-Henriksson H. Insulin-stimulated phosphorylation of the Akt substrate AS160 is impaired in skeletal muscle of type 2 diabetic subjects. Diabetes 2005; 54(6): 1692-7.
[http://dx.doi.org/10.2337/diabetes.54.6.1692] [PMID: 15919790]

[39]   Ramos PA, Lytle KA, Delivanis D, Nielsen S, LeBrasseur NK, Jensen MD. Insulin-stimulated muscle glucose uptake and insulin signaling in lean and obese humans. J Clin Endocrinol Metab 2021; 106(4): 1631-46.
[http://dx.doi.org/10.1210/clinem/dgaa919] [PMID: 33382888]

[40]   Lan ZJ, Lei Z, Nation L, *et al.* Oral administration of NPC43 counters hyperglycemia and activates insulin receptor in streptozotocin-induced type 1 diabetic mice. BMJ Open Diabetes Res Care 2020; 8(1): e001695.
[http://dx.doi.org/10.1136/bmjdrc-2020-001695] [PMID: 32998869]

[41]   Sakamoto K, Holman GD. Emerging role for AS160/TBC1D4 and TBC1D1 in the regulation of GLUT4 traffic. Am J Physiol Endocrinol Metab 2008; 295(1): E29-37.
[http://dx.doi.org/10.1152/ajpendo.90331.2008] [PMID: 18477703]

[42]   An D, Toyoda T, Taylor EB, *et al.* TBC1D1 regulates insulin- and contraction-induced glucose transport in mouse skeletal muscle. Diabetes 2010; 59(6): 1358-65.
[http://dx.doi.org/10.2337/db09-1266] [PMID: 20299473]

[43]   Giraldo PT. [Cardiovascular effects of an intensive intervention on lifestyle in type 2 diabetes]. Rev Clin Esp (Barc) 2014; 214(2): 102. [Cardiovascular effects of an intensive intervention on lifestyle in type 2 diabetes].
[PMID: 24772473]

[44]   Rejeski WJ, Bray GA, Chen SH, *et al.* Aging and physical function in type 2 diabetes: 8 years of an intensive lifestyle intervention. J Gerontol A Biol Sci Med Sci 2015; 70(3): 345-53.
[http://dx.doi.org/10.1093/gerona/glu083] [PMID: 24986062]

[45]   Richter EA, Kristiansen S, Wojtaszewski J, *et al.* Training effects on muscle glucose transport during exercise. Adv Exp Med Biol 1998; 441: 107-16.
[http://dx.doi.org/10.1007/978-1-4899-1928-1_10] [PMID: 9781318]

[46]   Martin IK, Katz A, Wahren J. Splanchnic and muscle metabolism during exercise in NIDDM patients. Am J Physiol 1995; 269(3 Pt 1): E583-90.
[PMID: 7573437]

[47]   Wojtaszewski JFP, Higaki Y, Hirshman MF, *et al.* Exercise modulates postreceptor insulin signaling and glucose transport in muscle-specific insulin receptor knockout mice. J Clin Invest 1999; 104(9): 1257-64.
[http://dx.doi.org/10.1172/JCI7961] [PMID: 10545524]

[48]   Stanford KI, Goodyear LJ. Exercise and type 2 diabetes: molecular mechanisms regulating glucose uptake in skeletal muscle. Adv Physiol Educ 2014; 38(4): 308-14.
[http://dx.doi.org/10.1152/advan.00080.2014] [PMID: 25434013]

[49]   Treebak JT, Glund S, Deshmukh A, *et al.* AMPK-mediated AS160 phosphorylation in skeletal muscle is dependent on AMPK catalytic and regulatory subunits. Diabetes 2006; 55(7): 2051-8.
[http://dx.doi.org/10.2337/db06-0175] [PMID: 16804075]

[50]   Funai K, Cartee GD. Contraction-stimulated glucose transport in rat skeletal muscle is sustained despite reversal of increased PAS-phosphorylation of AS160 and TBC1D1. J Appl Physiol 2008; 105(6): 1788-95.
[http://dx.doi.org/10.1152/japplphysiol.90838.2008] [PMID: 18818383]

[51]   Zisman A, Peroni OD, Abel ED, *et al.* Targeted disruption of the glucose transporter 4 selectively in muscle causes insulin resistance and glucose intolerance. Nat Med 2000; 6(8): 924-8.
[http://dx.doi.org/10.1038/78693] [PMID: 10932232]

[52]   Richter EA, Mikines KJ, Galbo H, Kiens B. Effect of exercise on insulin action in human skeletal muscle. J Appl Physiol 1989; 66(2): 876-85.
[http://dx.doi.org/10.1152/jappl.1989.66.2.876] [PMID: 2496078]

[53]   Dela F, Mikines KJ, von Linstow M, Secher NH, Galbo H. Effect of training on insulin-mediated glucose uptake in human muscle. Am J Physiol 1992; 263(6): E1134-43.
[PMID: 1476187]

[54]   Minuk HL, Vranic M, Marliss EB, Hanna AK, Albisser AM, Zinman B. Glucoregulatory and metabolic response to exercise in obese noninsulin-dependent diabetes. Am J Physiol 1981; 240(5): E458-64.
[PMID: 7015876]

[55]   O'Neill CC, Locke EJ, Sipf DA, *et al.* The effects of exercise training on glucose homeostasis and muscle metabolism in type 1 diabetic female mice. Metabolites 2022; 12(10): 948.
[http://dx.doi.org/10.3390/metabo12100948] [PMID: 36295850]

[56]   Andersen OE, Nielsen OB, Overgaard K. Early effects of eccentric contractions on muscle glucose uptake. J Appl Physiol 2019; 126(2): 376-85.
[http://dx.doi.org/10.1152/japplphysiol.00388.2018] [PMID: 30543500]

[57]   Kristiansen S, Gade J, Wojtaszewski JFP, Kiens B, Richter EA. Glucose uptake is increased in trained *vs.* untrained muscle during heavy exercise. J Appl Physiol 2000; 89(3): 1151-8.
[http://dx.doi.org/10.1152/jappl.2000.89.3.1151] [PMID: 10956363]

[58]   Joseph A, Parvathy S, Varma KK. Hyperinsulinemia induced altered insulin signaling pathway in muscle of high fat- and carbohydrate-fed rats: effect of exercise. J Diabetes Res 2021; 2021: 1-10.
[http://dx.doi.org/10.1155/2021/5123241] [PMID: 33708999]

[59]   Young JC, Kandarian SC, Kurowski TG. Skeletal muscle glucose uptake following overload-induced hypertrophy. Life Sci 1992; 50(18): 1319-25.
[http://dx.doi.org/10.1016/0024-3205(92)90282-T] [PMID: 1560731]

[60]   Sylow L, Kleinert M, Richter EA, Jensen TE. Exercise-stimulated glucose uptake — regulation and implications for glycaemic control. Nat Rev Endocrinol 2017; 13(3): 133-48.
[http://dx.doi.org/10.1038/nrendo.2016.162] [PMID: 27739515]

[61]   McMillin SL, Schmidt DL, Kahn BB, Witczak CA. GLUT4 is not necessary for overload-induced glucose uptake or hypertrophic growth in mouse skeletal muscle. Diabetes 2017; 66(6): 1491-500.
[http://dx.doi.org/10.2337/db16-1075] [PMID: 28279980]

[62]   McMillin SL, Evans PL, Taylor WM, *et al.* Muscle-specific ablation of glucose transporter 1 (GLUT1) does not impair basal or overload-stimulated skeletal muscle glucose uptake. Biomolecules 2022; 12(12): 1734.
[http://dx.doi.org/10.3390/biom12121734] [PMID: 36551162]

[63]   Mu J, Brozinick JT Jr, Valladares O, Bucan M, Birnbaum MJ. A role for AMP-activated protein kinase in contraction- and hypoxia-regulated glucose transport in skeletal muscle. Mol Cell 2001; 7(5): 1085-94.
[http://dx.doi.org/10.1016/S1097-2765(01)00251-9] [PMID: 11389854]

[64]   Cokorinos EC, Delmore J, Reyes AR, *et al.* Activation of skeletal muscle ampk promotes glucose disposal and glucose lowering in non-human primates and mice. Cell Metab 2017; 25(5): 1147-1159.e10.
[http://dx.doi.org/10.1016/j.cmet.2017.04.010] [PMID: 28467931]

[65]   Zhou G, Myers R, Li Y, *et al.* Role of AMP-activated protein kinase in mechanism of metformin action. J Clin Invest 2001; 108(8): 1167-74.
[http://dx.doi.org/10.1172/JCI13505] [PMID: 11602624]

[66]   Garbarino J, Sturley SL. Saturated with fat: new perspectives on lipotoxicity. Curr Opin Clin Nutr Metab Care 2009; 12(2): 110-6.
[http://dx.doi.org/10.1097/MCO.0b013e32832182ee] [PMID: 19202381]

[67]   Mahfouz R, Khoury R, Blachnio-Zabielska A, *et al.* Characterising the inhibitory actions of ceramide upon insulin signaling in different skeletal muscle cell models: a mechanistic insight. PLoS One 2014; 9(7): e101865.
[http://dx.doi.org/10.1371/journal.pone.0101865] [PMID: 25058613]

[68]   Kirwan JP. Plasma ceramides target skeletal muscle in type 2 diabetes. Diabetes 2013; 62(2): 352-4.
[http://dx.doi.org/10.2337/db12-1427] [PMID: 23349544]

[69]   Laurila PP, Wohlwend M, Imamura de Lima T, *et al.* Sphingolipids accumulate in aged muscle, and their reduction counteracts sarcopenia. Nature Aging 2022; 2(12): 1159-75.
[http://dx.doi.org/10.1038/s43587-022-00309-6] [PMID: 37118545]

[70]   Choi S, Snider AJ. Sphingolipids in high fat diet and obesity-related diseases. Mediators Inflamm 2015; 2015(1): 520618.
[http://dx.doi.org/10.1155/2015/520618] [PMID: 26648664]

[71]   Qi Y, Chen J, Lay A, Don A, Vadas M, Xia P. Loss of sphingosine kinase 1 predisposes to the onset of diabetes *via* promoting pancreatic β-cell death in diet-induced obese mice. FASEB J 2013; 27(10): 4294-304.
[http://dx.doi.org/10.1096/fj.13-230052] [PMID: 23839933]

[72]   Turner N, Kowalski GM, Leslie SJ, *et al.* Distinct patterns of tissue-specific lipid accumulation during the induction of insulin resistance in mice by high-fat feeding. Diabetologia 2013; 56(7): 1638-48.
[http://dx.doi.org/10.1007/s00125-013-2913-1] [PMID: 23620060]

[73]   Kajita K, Ishii I, Mori I, Asano M, Fuwa M, Morita H. Sphingosine 1-phosphate regulates obesity and glucose homeostasis. Int J Mol Sci 2024; 25(2): 932.
[http://dx.doi.org/10.3390/ijms25020932] [PMID: 38256005]

[74]   Ferrara PJ, Rong X, Maschek JA, *et al.* Lysophospholipid acylation modulates plasma membrane lipid organization and insulin sensitivity in skeletal muscle. J Clin Invest 2021; 131(8): e135963.
[http://dx.doi.org/10.1172/JCI135963] [PMID: 33591957]

[75]   Hilvo M, Meikle PJ, Pedersen ER, *et al.* Development and validation of a ceramide- and phospholipid-based cardiovascular risk estimation score for coronary artery disease patients. Eur Heart J 2020; 41(3): 371-80.
[http://dx.doi.org/10.1093/eurheartj/ehz387] [PMID: 31209498]

[76]   Mundra PA, Barlow CK, Nestel PJ, *et al.* Large-scale plasma lipidomic profiling identifies lipids that

predict cardiovascular events in secondary prevention. JCI Insight 2018; 3(17): e121326.
[http://dx.doi.org/10.1172/jci.insight.121326] [PMID: 30185661]

[77]   Tarasov K, Ekroos K, Suoniemi M, *et al.* Molecular lipids identify cardiovascular risk and are efficiently lowered by simvastatin and PCSK9 deficiency. J Clin Endocrinol Metab 2014; 99(1): E45-52.
[http://dx.doi.org/10.1210/jc.2013-2559] [PMID: 24243630]

[78]   Sigruener A, Kleber ME, Heimerl S, Liebisch G, Schmitz G, Maerz W. Glycerophospholipid and sphingolipid species and mortality: the Ludwigshafen Risk and Cardiovascular Health (LURIC) study. PLoS One 2014; 9(1): e85724.
[http://dx.doi.org/10.1371/journal.pone.0085724] [PMID: 24465667]

[79]   Tsalouhidou S, Argyrou C, Theofilidis G, *et al.* Mitochondrial phospholipids of rat skeletal muscle are less polyunsaturated than whole tissue phospholipids: Implications for protection against oxidative stress1. J Anim Sci 2006; 84(10): 2818-25.
[http://dx.doi.org/10.2527/jas.2006-031] [PMID: 16971584]

[80]   Adamson SE, Adak S, Petersen MC, *et al.* Decreased sarcoplasmic reticulum phospholipids in human skeletal muscle are associated with metabolic syndrome. J Lipid Res 2024; 65(3): 100519.
[http://dx.doi.org/10.1016/j.jlr.2024.100519] [PMID: 38354857]

[81]   Lee S, Norheim F, Gulseth HL, *et al.* Skeletal muscle phosphatidylcholine and phosphatidylethanolamine respond to exercise and influence insulin sensitivity in men. Sci Rep 2018; 8(1): 6531.
[http://dx.doi.org/10.1038/s41598-018-24976-x] [PMID: 29695812]

[82]   Verkerke ARP, Ferrara PJ, Lin CT, *et al.* Phospholipid methylation regulates muscle metabolic rate through Ca^{2+} transport efficiency. Nat Metab 2019; 1(9): 876-85.
[http://dx.doi.org/10.1038/s42255-019-0111-2] [PMID: 32405618]

[83]   Maurya SK, Herrera JL, Sahoo SK, *et al.* Sarcolipin signaling promotes mitochondrial biogenesis and oxidative metabolism in skeletal muscle. Cell Rep 2018; 24(11): 2919-31.
[http://dx.doi.org/10.1016/j.celrep.2018.08.036] [PMID: 30208317]

[84]   Gamu D, Trinh A, Bombardier E, Tupling AR. Persistence of diet-induced obesity despite access to voluntary activity in mice lacking sarcolipin. Physiol Rep 2015; 3(9): e12549.
[http://dx.doi.org/10.14814/phy2.12549] [PMID: 26400985]

[85]   Bal NC, Maurya SK, Sopariwala DH, *et al.* Sarcolipin is a newly identified regulator of muscle-based thermogenesis in mammals. Nat Med 2012; 18(10): 1575-9.
[http://dx.doi.org/10.1038/nm.2897] [PMID: 22961106]

[86]   Mascioni A, Karim C, Barany G, Thomas DD, Veglia G. Structure and orientation of sarcolipin in lipid environments. Biochemistry 2002; 41(2): 475-82.
[http://dx.doi.org/10.1021/bi011243m] [PMID: 11781085]

CHAPTER 2

The Role of Skeletal Muscles in Metabolic Dysfunction-Associated Steatotic Liver Disease

Ikuru Miura[1,*]

[1] *Faculty of Sports and Health Science, Fukuoka University, Fukuoka, Japan*

Abstract: Skeletal muscles and the liver share functions as metabolic organs, and there are known crosstalk in their pathophysiology. In today's world, where obesity is rampant, many people suffer from metabolic abnormalities associated with obesity, posing a global health issue. This chapter summarizes the latest findings on the crosstalk between metabolic dysfunction-associated steatotic liver disease (MASLD) and skeletal muscles, which starts and progresses in association with obesity and its associated systemic metabolic abnormalities.

Keywords: Muscle-Liver axis, MAFLD/MASH, NAFLD/NASH, Skeletal muscle.

INTRODUCTION

Skeletal muscles are the largest organs in the body, and they have roles in locomotor function and metabolism of glucose and lipids. They also act as endocrine organs, secreting bioactive substances known as myokine. Decreases in muscle mass, such as sarcopenia and metabolic dysfunction, are associated with numerous diseases, including type 2 diabetes, lipid disorders, metabolic dysfunction-associated steatotic liver disease (MASLD), and cognitive impairment, among others [1 - 3]. The skeletal muscle and liver share functions as metabolic organs, contributing to systemic metabolic regulation through mutual cooperation (Muscle-Liver axis). There is a crosstalk between the dysfunction and pathology of skeletal muscle and liver. Regarding this pathophysiological crosstalk, it may be easy to understand that when dysfunction occurs in one organ, the other organ alone must process the same function, placing a significant burden on that organ. This chapter summarizes the relationship between quantitative and qualitative changes in skeletal muscle and the pathophysiology of MASLD, as

---

[*] **Corresponding author Ikuru Miura:** Faculty of Sports and Health Science, Fukuoka University, Fukuoka, Japan; E-mail: miurai@fukuoka-u.ac.jp

Hiroaki Eshima, Ikuru Miura, Yutaka Matsunaga & Yuki Tomiga (Eds.)

well as introduces the mediators of the muscle-liver axis that have been elucidated thus far.

It should be noted that MASLD is a newly defined concept of a disease introduced in 2023, which redefines previously known conditions such as nonalcoholic fatty liver disease (NAFLD) or metabolic dysfunction-associated fatty liver disease (MAFLD). First, I will briefly outline the definitions, name changes, and the process of redefinition for each condition. However, evidence and reviews mentioning MASLD are limited to date. Unless otherwise specified, I will treat these conditions in the chapter as synonymous. However, since the definition of each disease is strictly different, the names of the diseases used in the original texts are used when referring to previous studies.

DEFINITION OF METABOLIC DYSFUNCTION-ASSOCIATED STEATOTIC LIVER DISEASE (MASLD)

It is known that overweight and obesity induce fat deposition in the liver, which in turn leads to hepatic inflammation and fibrosis. Hepatic inflammation and fibrosis can lead to more serious diseases such as cirrhosis and hepatocellular carcinoma, and their pathogenesis has been attracting attention with the increase in the obese population. Hepatic inflammation and fibrosis based on the fatty liver caused by obesity or overweight were first reported and named "non-alcoholic steatohepatitis (NASH) " by Jurgen Ludwing in 1980. The term "non-alcoholic fatty liver disease (NAFLD) is used to distinguish non-alcoholic fatty liver (NAFL), which is a benign fatty liver that shows lipid deposits in the liver from NASH, and to describe the progression of the disease from NALF to NASH. NAFLD is used as a disease concept to describe a chronic liver disease that progresses to hepatitis and fibrosis with systemic metabolic abnormalities based on obesity and ectopic fat deposition in the liver without a clear history of alcohol consumption (less than 30g/day in men and 20g/day in women in terms of ethanol). In today's society, the number of obese people continues to increase, and the number of patients with NAFLD is also growing worldwide. It is recognized as one of the most common chronic liver diseases [4, 5].

NAFLD presents two distinct conditions: benign NAFL and malignant NASH. In addition, given that liver biopsy is required for definitive diagnosis, it is unsuitable for the efficient screening of high-risk fatty liver patients in clinical practice. There is also a concern that the relatively low alcohol intake standard may exclude patients with a drinking habit. Therefore, a new disease concept focusing on metabolic abnormalities involved in the progression from fatty liver to hepatitis and fibrosis, "Metabolic dysfunction-associated fatty liver disease (MAFLD)", was proposed in 2020. In addition to fatty liver, MAFLD is defined by the presence of obesity or type 2 diabetes or meeting two or more criteria indicating abnormalities in glucose or lipid metabolism. As mentioned above, although NAFLD and MAFLD have different diagnostic criteria, they represent concepts that are shared by many patients in reality. However, when comparing MAFLD with NAFLD, MAFLD allows for the exclusion of low-risk fatty liver patients without metabolic abnormalities while identifying high-risk fatty liver patients with metabolic abnormalities and a history of alcohol consumption. Additionally, since liver biopsy is not required for diagnosis, MAFLD was expected to be a useful disease concept for screening high-risk fatty liver patients. However, many people are resistant to the terms "alcoholic" and "fatty" used in NAFLD and MAFLD, and the problem that there is a group of patients who are excluded from screening in NAFLD and MAFLD remains unresolved. There have always been calls by medical doctors and medical researchers toredefine the disease concept.

Against this background, efforts were made to create a new concept of the disease in 2023 through the cooperation of institutions around the world, led by the American Association for the Study of Liver Disease (AASLD) and the European Association for the Study of the Liver (EASL) [6]. The concept of steatotic liver disease (SLD) was proposed as a generic term for fatty liver diseases of various etiologies. These are classified into five categories according to pathogenesis and cause. The concept of MASLD was proposed as a concept similar to the conventional NAFLD or MASLD. MASLD was defined as a fatty liver with an abnormal level of one or more of the following cardiometabolic risk factors (BNI or waist diameter), abnormal glucose metabolism (blood glucose level or HbA1C), blood pressure, blood triglycerides, and blood HDL cholesterol (Fig. **1**). In addition, metabolic dysfunction-associated steatohepatitis (MASH) was also proposed as an alternative to conventional NASH. Although MASLD/MASH is expected to replace NAFLD/NASH or MAFLD in clinical practice in the future, it would be more meaningful to treat these disease concepts as synonymous to some extent for the time being in terms of accumulation of scientific knowledge.

MECHANISM OF ONSET AND PROGRESSION OF NASH (MASH): THE MULTIPLE PARALLEL HITS HYPOTHESIS

Although NASH is a serious liver disease that can progress to cirrhosis and hepatocellular carcinoma, there are few preventive and curative measures to date. One reason for this is the complexity of the pathogenesis and progression mechanism. "The multiple parallel hits hypothesis" proposed in 2010 is supported as a mechanism for the onset and progression of NASH [7, 8]. This hypothesis suggests that multiple extrahepatic organ abnormalities are involved in the onset and progression of NASH in parallel hits.

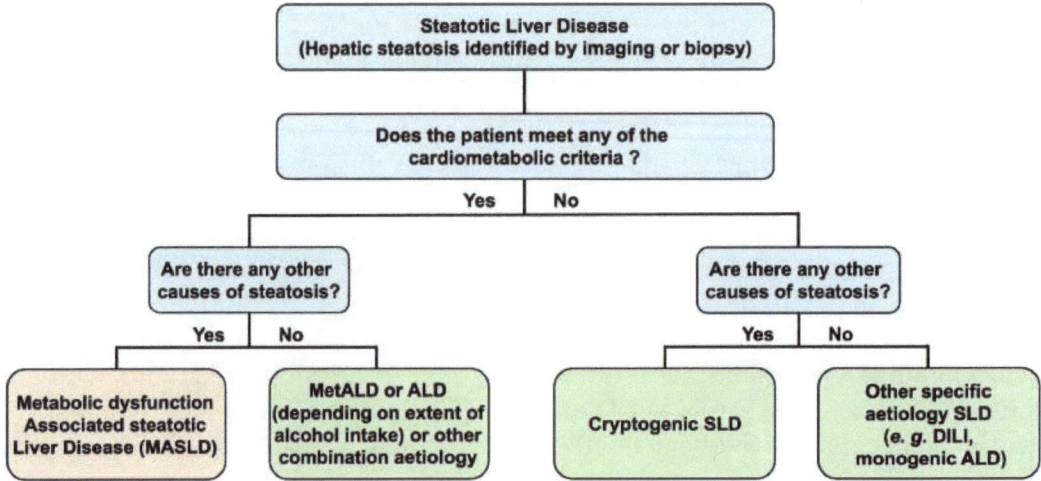

Fig. (1). Flowchart of MASLD diagnosis prepared by the author based on reference [6].

In this multiple parallel hit hypothesis, it has been shown that hepatic inflammation caused by excessive influx of lipopolysaccharide (LPS), a bacterial component of the intestinal microbiota, resulting from alterations in the intestinal microbiota and increased intestinal permeability, plays an important role in the onset and progression of NASH (Gut-Liver axis). In addition, the secretion of hormones and inflammatory cytokines from visceral adipose tissue accumulated in excess as a result of obesity and excessive influx of free fatty acid into the liver have been implicated (Adipose tissue-liver axis). Other factors, such as age-related muscle atrophy (sarcopenia) and insulin resistance in skeletal muscle, also contribute to the onset and progression of NASH (Muscle-liver axis) [2]. Thus, since the multiple parallel hits hypothesis was proposed, NASH has been recognized as an obesity-based systemic disease. In this chapter, I will focus on the relationship between MASLD and skeletal muscle pathology and the mechanism of the muscle-liver axis.

Relationship of Skeletal Muscle Mass and MASLD

In skeletal muscle, muscle protein synthesis and breaking down are constant, and the balance between the two determines skeletal muscle mass. In other words, skeletal muscle mass decreases when the rate of muscle protein breaking down exceeds the rate of synthesis. Factors that induce skeletal muscle atrophy include energy deficiency (fasting), physical inactivity, aging, and cachexia [9 - 12]. MASLD is a disease exacerbated by muscle mass loss. Since MASLD is more common in middle-aged and elderly patients, it has been reported to be associated with sarcopenia, an age-related muscle atrophy [2].

In a seven-year cohort study on more than 10,000 subjects, populations with lower skeletal muscle index [SMI: limb skeletal muscle/body weight (%)], an index of skeletal mass at baseline, had a higher incidence of NAFLD during follow-up [13]. In addition, skeletal muscle atrophy develops earlier in patients with severe NAFLD compared to those with mild NAFLD [14]. In a study examining the association between sarcopenia and NASH using liver biopsy, a definitive diagnostic method for NASH [15], sarcopenia was shown to be associated with NASH pathogenesis, especially hepatic fibrosis, independently of BMI, metabolic abnormalities (insulin resistance), and other factors. In a large prospective cohort study of approximately 330,000 subjects [16], low skeletal muscle mass was also shown to be associated with the development of NAFLD.

Obesity, as well as sarcopenia, plays a major role in the onset and progression of MASLD. In a quartile analysis performed by our group using the index sarcopenia obesity [quartiles into which their skeletal muscle mass to visceral fat area ratio: SV ratio (g/cm^2)], the group with the lowest SV ratio was found to have a greater accumulation of hepatic steatosis and more severe inflammation [17]. In addition, the concentration of urinary titin-N-fragment, a maker of skeletal muscle catabolism, increased with the progression of liver lesions [18]. These previous studies indicate a close relationship between sarcopenia and MASLD pathological progression, suggesting that maintenance of skeletal muscle mass may prevent the progression of MASLD.

Many studies, including the previous studies mentioned above, have used indices of skeletal muscle mass that normalize muscle mass for body weight. Since obese persons have naturally high body weights, there is a risk of estimating skeletal muscle lower than it should be when skeletal muscle mass indices that include body weight or BMI are used. Indeed, cohort studies using an index of skeletal muscle mass normalized by height have reported that reduced skeletal muscle mass decreases the risk of NAFLD [19]. This discrepancy may be because, to date, no definition of skeletal muscle loss or sarcopenia has been established for patients with MASLD. When discussing the relationship between skeletal muscle mass and MASLD pathophysiology, attention should be paid to the index of skeletal muscle mass and its definition.

Skeletal muscle in patients with MASLD is now being assessed in more detail, and in addition to muscle mass, composition is also being evaluated. Interestingly, a report showed that myosteatosis, a decrease in myofiber density due to fat deposition, may be a screening tool to clearly distinguish NAFL from NASH [20, 21]. In the same report [20], it was mentioned that patients who showed improvement in liver pathology following obesity intervention also showed improvement in myosteatosis. Thus, it is becoming clear that not only skeletal muscle weight but also changes in its composition are associated with MASLD pathology. Naturally, the question arises: how are changes in skeletal muscle mass and composition related to the development of MASLD? The answer to this question may be useful in the development of MASLD prevention methods. A prospective intervention study was conducted in an animal model [22]. This study showed that only mice with severe NASH showing hepatic fibrosis had reduced skeletal muscle mass (sarcopenia). In contrast, mice with early NASH, before hepatic fibrosis developed, did not onset sarcopenia. In addition, myosteatosis was found to occur earlier than sarcopenia as a skeletal muscle and myosteatosis, unlike sarcopenia, was found to be associated with the onset of early NASH. Based on the results of previous studies, myosteatosis is considered to occur at a relatively early stage and to be associated with the onset of NASH. However, the causal relationship between the deterioration of skeletal muscle composition, such as myosteatosis and liver lesions, and its mediating factor are not fully understood. Future research trends should be closely monitored.

Relationship of Skeletal Muscle Function and MASLD

Along with muscle mass, muscle weakness is an important factor in defining sarcopenia. Basically, skeletal muscle mass (cross-sectional area of muscle fibers) and muscle strength are proportional to each other. However, it is known that during the process of sarcopenia formation, muscle weakness precedes a decrease in muscle mass [23]. It is known that muscle weakness, as well as muscle mass loss, is associated with exacerbation of MAFLD pathology. In the prospective follow-up study described above, an association was found between the index of muscle strength (grip strength) and NAFLD severity [16]. Our group also reported that the decreased grip strength and knee extensor muscle strength are associated with NASH severity (hepatic inflammation and fibrosis) [18]. In addition, atherosclerotic cardiovascular disease (ASCVD) is known to be a major cause of death in MAFLD patients, and it has been reported that decreased grip strength in MAFLD patients increases the risk of developing and progressing to ASCVD [24].

Deterioration of physical function due to decreased muscle strength is also known to be associated with liver lesions. A report of a 6-minute walk test (measuring the distance that can be walked in 6 minutes) in patients with hepatitis B, hepatitis C, and cirrhosis revealed that poor walking function was associated with liver lesion progression and mortality, indicating that the 6-minutes walk test may be a useful prognostic indicator for life outcome in chronic liver disease [25]. Other reports have shown an association between decreased walking speed and worsening of liver lesions [25], suggesting that reduced muscle strength and deterioration of physical function may also promote the progression of liver lesions.

Loss of skeletal muscle mass and changes in muscle composition can be screening tools for MAFLD, but these accurate measurements require special equipment such as MRI. MASLD (NAFLD) is the most common chronic liver disease and is estimated to affect over 1 billion people worldwide [4, 5]. Considering the number of patients with MASLD, it is impractical to measure skeletal muscle mass and muscle composition in all patients due to the enormous cost involved. On the other hand, muscle strength and gait tests can be measured at relatively low prices regardless of location and are expected to be useful tools for screening patients with MASLD.

Skeletal muscles also function as metabolic organs. In particular, approximately 90% of insulin-mediated systemic glucose utilization occurs in skeletal muscle [26]. Maintenance of normal muscle function is important to maintain homeostasis of glucose metabolism. Obesity and physical inactivity induce insulin resistance in skeletal muscle [2, 26], and obesity-induced insulin resistance in patients is a major aggravating factor in MASLD. Obesity is also associated with increased oxidative stress and inflammation [27], and chronicity of these factors leads to abnormal skeletal muscle mitochondria. Dysfunction of muscle mitochondria attenuates fatty acid β-oxidation and induces fat deposition in muscle [28]. Deterioration of muscle composition is associated with exacerbation of MASLD pathology, suggesting that skeletal muscle metabolic abnormalities may accelerate the progression of liver lesions. The impact of skeletal muscle metabolic abnormalities on MASLD will be introduced in more detail later, but abnormalities in skeletal muscle function (muscle strength and metabolic function) are closely associated with the exacerbation of MASLD pathology.

MEDIATOR OF MUSCLE-LIVER AXIS

Since the existence of crosstalk between skeletal muscle and liver lesions (Muscle-Liver axis) was discovered through the accumulation of clinical studies, the mechanism and mediators of crosstalk have been investigated. The mediators of the muscle-liver axis in MASLD that have been elucidated to date will be introduced here (Fig. **2**).

Insulin Resistance (IR)

Dietary glucose is taken up by skeletal muscle and liver and stored as glycogen. Muscle glycogen is the main source of energy for muscle contraction and is used during sports and physical activity. The liver, unlike skeletal muscle, has a glucose-6-phospatase (G6Pase) that degrades glycogen to glucose, thus contributing to the maintenance of blood glucose levels by degrading glycogen to glucose and releasing it into the blood. Thus, skeletal muscle and liver cooperate with each other to control glucose metabolism in the whole body.

When glucose is taken into the body, insulin is secreted from the pancreas. Insulin acts on skeletal muscle and liver *via* the bloodstream and induces translocation of glucose transporters to the plasma membrane through intracellular signaling to bring blood glucose into the cells. Glucose transporter 4 (GLUT4) is expressed mainly in skeletal muscle, and glucose transporter 2 (GLUT2) is expressed in the liver [29]. Since glucose alone cannot pass through the cell membrane, the cooperation of insulin-glucose transporter is essential for blood glucose uptake. When intracellular signaling by insulin is weakened for some reason, and the translocation of glucose transporter is inhibited, blood glucose uptake by insulin is reduced. This condition is called insulin resistance (IR) and is recognized as a pathological condition underlying metabolic diseases such as T2DM and MASLD.

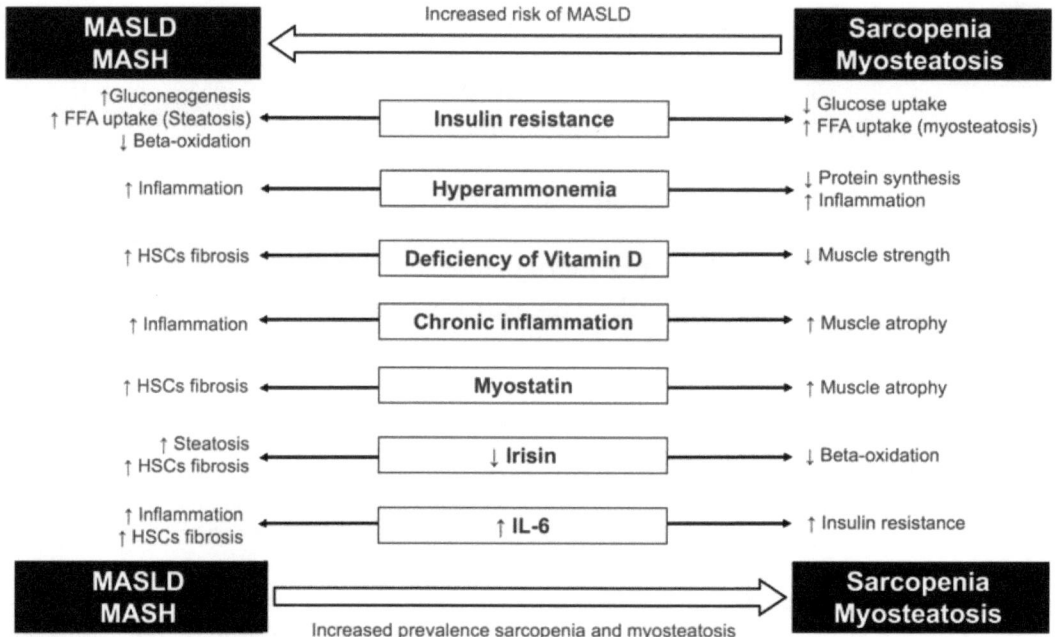

Fig. (2). Mediators of muscle-liver axis in MASLD modified by the author based on reference [2].

Obesity is a risk factor for the induction of skeletal muscle IR. In obese individuals, excessive visceral fat accumulation causes the secretion of inflammatory cytokines from adipose tissue, which induces inflammation in skeletal muscle, resulting in IR [30]. It has also been suggested that obesity causes ectopic fat deposition in skeletal muscle (myosteatosis), which may induce IR [31]. Since skeletal muscle is the largest glucose-processing organ in the body, the formation of IR in skeletal muscle leads to the disruption of systemic glucose homeostasis.

There is a close association between IR and MASLD pathogenesis, with an approximately 5-fold increased prevalence of NAFLD in T2DM patients with abnormal glucose metabolism compared to non-T2DM patients [32]. In the IR state, glucose utilization is suppressed, resulting in increased lipolysis in adipose tissue and increased free fatty acid concentration in the blood, which then flows into the liver. Excess fatty acid influx to the liver leads to triglyceride (TG) accumulation, resulting in the progression of hepatic steatosis [33]. Fatty acids such as palmitic acid are toxic (lipotoxicity) and promote NASH by inducing inflammation, oxidant stress, and endoplasmic reticulum (ER) stress in the liver, causing cell death [34]. In addition, the inhibition of glycogen degradation by insulin is inhibited in IR, resulting in increased glucose neogenesis in the liver despite hyperglycemia. Excess glucose leads to the production of advanced glycation end-products (AGEs), which induce the formation of reactive oxidative species (ROSs), an enhanced inflammatory response, and activation of hepatic stellate cells (HSCs), promoting hepatic inflammation and fibrosis [35]. It has also been pointed out that increased glucose neogenesis in the liver promotes proteolysis, which may induce the formation of sarcopenia [36]. Thus, obesity-based IR is a common pathological factor for MASLD and sarcopenia and is a central mediator of the muscle-liver axis.

Hyperammonemia

In MASLD and cirrhosis, the urea cycle in the liver is abnormal, resulting in hyperammonemia. Hyperammonemia is a risk factor for sarcopenia. Ammonia suppressed mechanistic target of rapamycin (mTOR) complex1 (mTORC1) signaling, a positive regulator of muscle protein synthesis, *via* activation of general control non-depressible 2 (GCN2) in skeletal muscle and promotes muscle atrophy by attenuating muscle protein synthesis [37]. In addition, branched-chain amino acids (BCAAs) have the ability to stimulate muscle protein synthesis, but in conditions of hyperammonemia, BCAAs are consumed to metabolize ammonia in skeletal muscle [37].

Metabolic adaptations of skeletal muscle also occur in response to hyperammonemia. In hyperammonemia, ammonia concentrations in skeletal muscle are markedly increased, which enhances the metabolic pathway that produces glutamate from ammonia and α-ketoglutarate [38]. α-ketoglutarate is an intermediate metabolite of the TCA cycle, and its accumulation may lead to slowing of the TCA cycle, abnormal function of mitochondria, and decreased ATP production. Since protein synthesis requires a large amount of energy, a decrease in ATP levels may reduce muscle protein synthesis.

Ammonia activates nuclear factor kappa B (NF-kB), a major inflammatory transcription factor, and increases the expression of myostatin /GDF-8, a factor that promotes muscle atrophy [39]. Clinical studies on patients with cirrhosis reported a positive correlation between blood ammonia level and myostatin level and a negative correlation between blood ammonia level and BCAA level [40].

Deficiency of Vitamin D

Patients with NAFLD have decreased blood vitamin D levels [41, 42], suggesting that vitamin D deficiency is involved in the progression of MASLD. It has been shown that the expression of vitamin D receptor (VDR) in liver tissue is concentrated in non-parenchymal cells such as HSCs [43]. The activation of HSCs induces hepatic fibrosis, and it has been reported that the interaction of VDR ligands and VDR to inhibit Tgf-β1/SMAD signaling may suppress hepatic fibrosis[43]. Vitamin D has also been found to regulate the expression of the insulin receptor in insulin-target organs, including the liver [44], and its formation of insulin resistance by vitamin D deficiency may also be involved in the progression of liver lesions.

Vitamin D and VDR have also been shown to be involved in the regulation of skeletal muscle mass and function. Vitamin D is involved in myoblast proliferation and differentiation and may play an important role in skeletal muscle formation [45]. In fact, it has been reported that blood vitamin D levels decrease in populations with sarcopenia, similar to those of MASLD patients [36]. Vitamin D is also involved in skeletal muscle function, and its deficiency is associated with muscle weakness [46]. As described above, there is accumulating evidence that vitamin D deficiency is involved in the progression of liver and skeletal muscle lesions.

Chronic Inflammation

Chronic inflammation is a common pathogenetic basis for MASLD and sarcopenia. Although there are multiple pathways for obesity-induced inflammation, its mechanism is introduced in accordance with the "multiple parallel hits hypothesis" for the onset and progression of NASH. In obese individuals, lipopolysaccharides (LPS), a bacterial component of intestinal bacteria, easily flow into the blood from the intestinal tract due to the transformation of microbiota and increased intestinal permeability (leaky gut) following overeating, overnutrition, and high-fat diet, resulting in metabolic endotoxemia [47]. LPS entering the liver from the intestinal tract *via* the portal vein is recognized as foreign *via* toll-like receptor 4 (TLR4) by immune cells, including Kupffer cells, which are tissue macrophages of the liver, and induces hepatic inflammation by activating inflammatory signals [34]. In NAFLD patients, hepatic LPS clearance is decreased [17], which may lead to prolonged LPS retention time in the liver and chronic inflammation. Under the condition of chronic inflammation, immune cells (*e.g.*, macrophage) secrete large amounts of inflammatory cytokines such as tumor necrosis factor-α and interleukin-1β (Il-1β). At the same time, the generation of ROSs increases, inducing oxidative stress. The expression of factors that induce activation of HSCs, such as transforming growth factor β1 (Tgf-β1), and induce hepatic fibrosis also increases under conditions of inflammation and oxidative stress. Choric inflammation and oxidative stress in the liver are involved in IR and cell death and are closely related to the severity of hepatic inflammation and fibrosis. LPS-induced inflammation has also been shown to be involved in muscle atrophy and skeletal muscle formation [48, 49]. In *in vitro* experiment, it has been shown that the addition of LPS inhibits myoblast to myotube formation [48, 49]. It has been suggested that the activation of NF-kB may be involved as a mechanism. In addition, it has been confirmed that administration of LPS causes inflammation in muscle cells, resulting in myofiber atrophy [48, 49]. On the other hand, the administration of an inhibitor of TLR4, the receptor for LPS, has been shown to completely suppress LPS-induced myofiber atrophy. Liver and skeletal muscle dysfunction exacerbate each other's disease states. Metabolic endotoxemia associated with obese individuals is an important pathological factor involved in both liver and skeletal muscle.

Myokine

Skeletal muscle cells secrete bioactive substances called myokines [50], which exert various effects on other organs *via* blood flow. Several myokines have been found to affect hepatic pathology. Three major myokines were introduced here, which are widely recognized to affect MASLD.

Myostatin/GDF-8

Myostatin is a secreted protein belonging to the Tgf-β family and is known to have potent muscle atrophy effects. Myostatin-deficient mice have been reported to show a dramatic increase in skeletal muscle mass [51]. Myostatin is involved in the major muscle atrophy pathway, ubiquitin-proteasome, and autophagy and plays an important role as a negative regulator of muscle mass [52]. It has also been shown that blood myostatin levels are increased in patients with cirrhosis [53], and a relationship with liver disease has also been reported. In a study on patients with cirrhosis, it was reported that increased blood myostatin levels were associated with decreased skeletal muscle mass and survival [40]. Myostatin exerts its function *via* activin receptor 2B (Acvr2b), and it has been reported that Acvr2b is expressed in HSCs [54]. Furthermore, *in vivo* experiments have shown that myostatin activates HSCs *via* Acvr2b and induces hepatic fibrosis [55]. Myostatin may not only induce skeletal muscle atrophy and indirectly contribute to the progression of liver lesions but may also directly induce the progression of hepatic fibrosis.

Irisin

Irisin is a myokine that is cleaved from fibronectin type 2 domain-containing protein 5 (FNDC5) and released into the extracellular. Its main function is to induce browning of white adipose tissue and increase heat production and energy expenditure [56]. In patients with advanced hepatic steatosis, blood irisin levels are decreased, suggesting that irisin suppresses hepatic steatosis [57]. *in vitro* experiments suggest that irisin may inhibit fat deposition in hepatocytes by suppressing the activity of transcription factors involved in lipid synthesis [58, 59]. Defects in FNDC5 have also been shown to cause severe hepatic fibrosis *via* activation of HSCs [60]. Irisin secretion is regulated by peroxisome proliferator-activated receptor γ coactivator-1α (PGC-1α) [58]. It is known that exercise and physical activity increase irisin secretion [61]. Increasing irisin secretion from skeletal muscle cells may be important for the prevention and treatment of MASLD *via* the muscle-liver axis.

Interleukin-6 (IL-6)

IL-6, the earliest myokine identified[50], is known to have both pro- and anti-inflammatory function [62]. In patients with NAFLD, blood IL-6 levels have been shown to increase [63], and its relevance to the disease has been recognized. In *in vivo* experiments, it has been shown that administration of a high dose of IL-6 induces muscle atrophy [64]. It has also been reported that IL-6 induces obesity-associated IR formation [65]. IL-6 secreted from skeletal muscle may act paracrinely on neighboring muscle cells and induce IR formation that exacerbates MASLD pathology.

Exercise contributes to the improvement of IR in skeletal muscle, and it has been suggested that IL-6 secreted from muscle cells during exercise may suppress the expression of other inflammatory cytokines and inhibit inflammation in skeletal muscles [66]. IL-6 is myokine with multiple functions and pro- and anti-inflammatory disorders of organs. Further studies are needed to elucidate its complex functions.

CONCLUSION

To elucidate the pathogenesis of MASLD, a systemic metabolic disease based on obesity, a research approach from an organ-crosstalk perspective is required.

Skeletal muscles share multiple functions with the liver, and it has been shown that there is a close crosstalk in the pathogenesis of MASLD. Elucidating the role of skeletal muscle in MASLD will help establish evidence-based prevention and treatment for MASLD, for which there is still no fundamental prevention or treatment. However, the mechanism of the muscle-liver axis and its mediators remain unclear. Elucidation of these factors is needed to elucidate the pathogenesis of MASLD and identify prevention and treatment methods.

REFFERNCES

[1]   Hong S, Chang Y, Jung HS, Yun KE, Shin H, Ryu S. Relative muscle mass and the risk of incident type 2 diabetes: A cohort study. PLoS One 2017; 12(11): e0188650.
[http://dx.doi.org/10.1371/journal.pone.0188650] [PMID: 29190709]

[2]   Bhanji RA, Narayanan P, Allen AM, Malhi H, Watt KD. Sarcopenia in hiding: The risk and consequence of underestimating muscle dysfunction in nonalcoholic steatohepatitis. Hepatology 2017; 66(6): 2055-65.
[http://dx.doi.org/10.1002/hep.29420] [PMID: 28777879]

[3]   Severinsen MCK, Pedersen BK. Muscle–organ crosstalk: the emerging roles of myokines. Endocr Rev 2020; 41(4): 594-609.
[http://dx.doi.org/10.1210/endrev/bnaa016] [PMID: 32393961]

[4]   Loomba R, Friedman SL, Shulman GI. Mechanisms and disease consequences of nonalcoholic fatty liver disease. Cell 2021; 184(10): 2537-64.
[http://dx.doi.org/10.1016/j.cell.2021.04.015] [PMID: 33989548]

[5]   Younossi ZM. Non-alcoholic fatty liver disease – A global public health perspective. J Hepatol 2019; 70(3): 531-44.
[http://dx.doi.org/10.1016/j.jhep.2018.10.033] [PMID: 30414863]

[6]   Rinella ME, Lazarus JV, Ratziu V, *et al.* A multisociety Delphi consensus statement on new fatty liver disease nomenclature. J Hepatol 2023; 79(6): 1542-56.
[http://dx.doi.org/10.1016/j.jhep.2023.06.003] [PMID: 37364790]

[7]   Tilg H, Moschen AR. Evolution of inflammation in nonalcoholic fatty liver disease: The multiple parallel hits hypothesis. Hepatology 2010; 52(5): 1836-46.
[http://dx.doi.org/10.1002/hep.24001] [PMID: 21038418]

[8]   Tilg H, Adolph TE, Moschen AR. Multiple parallel hits hypothesis in nonalcoholic fatty liver disease: revisited after a decade. Hepatology 2021; 73(2): 833-42.
[http://dx.doi.org/10.1002/hep.31518] [PMID: 32780879]

[9]   Pasiakos SM, Cao JJ, Margolis LM, *et al.* Effects of high-protein diets on fat-free mass and muscle protein synthesis following weight loss: a randomized controlled trial. FASEB J 2013; 27(9): 3837-47.
[http://dx.doi.org/10.1096/fj.13-230227] [PMID: 23739654]

[10]   Eggelbusch M, Charlton BT, Bosutti A, *et al.* The impact of bed rest on human skeletal muscle metabolism. Cell Rep Med 2024; 5(1): 101372.
[http://dx.doi.org/10.1016/j.xcrm.2023.101372] [PMID: 38232697]

[11]   Sayer AA, Cruz-Jentoft A. Sarcopenia definition, diagnosis and treatment: consensus is growing. Age Ageing 2022; 51(10): afac220.
[http://dx.doi.org/10.1093/ageing/afac220] [PMID: 36273495]

[12]   Dolly A, Dumas JF, Servais S. Cancer cachexia and skeletal muscle atrophy in clinical studies: what do we really know? J Cachexia Sarcopenia Muscle 2020; 11(6): 1413-28.
[http://dx.doi.org/10.1002/jcsm.12633] [PMID: 33053604]

[13]   Kim G, Lee SE, Lee YB, *et al.* Relationship between relative skeletal muscle mass and nonalcoholic fatty liver disease: A 7-year longitudinal study. Hepatology 2018; 68(5): 1755-68.
[http://dx.doi.org/10.1002/hep.30049] [PMID: 29679374]

[14]   Sinn DH, Kang D, Kang M, *et al.* Nonalcoholic fatty liver disease and accelerated loss of skeletal muscle mass: A longitudinal cohort study. Hepatology 2022; 76(6): 1746-54.
[http://dx.doi.org/10.1002/hep.32578] [PMID: 35588190]

[15]   Koo BK, Kim D, Joo SK, *et al.* Sarcopenia is an independent risk factor for non-alcoholic steatohepatitis and significant fibrosis. J Hepatol 2017; 66(1): 123-31.
[http://dx.doi.org/10.1016/j.jhep.2016.08.019] [PMID: 27599824]

[16]   Petermann-Rocha F, Gray SR, Forrest E, *et al.* Associations of muscle mass and grip strength with severe NAFLD: A prospective study of 333,295 UK Biobank participants. J Hepatol 2022; 76(5): 1021-9.
[http://dx.doi.org/10.1016/j.jhep.2022.01.010] [PMID: 35085594]

[17]   Shida T, Akiyama K, Oh S, *et al.* Skeletal muscle mass to visceral fat area ratio is an important determinant affecting hepatic conditions of non-alcoholic fatty liver disease. J Gastroenterol 2018; 53(4): 535-47.
[http://dx.doi.org/10.1007/s00535-017-1377-3] [PMID: 28791501]

[18]   Oshida N, Shida T, Oh S, *et al.* Urinary levels of titin-n fragment, a skeletal muscle damage marker, are increased in subjects with nonalcoholic fatty liver disease. Sci Rep 2019; 9(1): 19498.
[http://dx.doi.org/10.1038/s41598-019-56121-7] [PMID: 31862937]

[19]   Peng TC, Wu LW, Chen WL, Liaw FY, Chang YW, Kao TW. Nonalcoholic fatty liver disease and sarcopenia in a Western population (NHANES III): The importance of sarcopenia definition. Clin Nutr 2019; 38(1): 422-8.
[http://dx.doi.org/10.1016/j.clnu.2017.11.021] [PMID: 29287676]

[20]   Nachit M, Kwanten WJ, Thissen JP, *et al.* Muscle fat content is strongly associated with NASH: A longitudinal study in patients with morbid obesity. J Hepatol 2021; 75(2): 292-301.
[http://dx.doi.org/10.1016/j.jhep.2021.02.037] [PMID: 33865909]

[21]   Hsieh YC, Joo SK, Koo BK, *et al.* Myosteatosis, but not sarcopenia, predisposes nafld subjects to early steatohepatitis and fibrosis progression. Clin Gastroenterol Hepatol 2023; 21(2): 388-397.e10.
[http://dx.doi.org/10.1016/j.cgh.2022.01.020] [PMID: 35101634]

[22]   Nachit M, De Rudder M, Thissen JP, *et al.* Myosteatosis rather than sarcopenia associates with non-alcoholic steatohepatitis in non-alcoholic fatty liver disease preclinical models. J Cachexia Sarcopenia Muscle 2021; 12(1): 144-58.
[http://dx.doi.org/10.1002/jcsm.12646] [PMID: 33244884]

[23]   Goodpaster BH, Park SW, Harris TB, *et al.* The loss of skeletal muscle strength, mass, and quality in older adults: the health, aging and body composition study. J Gerontol A Biol Sci Med Sci 2006; 61(10): 1059-64.
[http://dx.doi.org/10.1093/gerona/61.10.1059] [PMID: 17077199]

[24]   Choi KY, Kim TY, Chon YE, *et al.* Impact of anthropometric parameters on outcomes in Asians with metabolic dysfunction-associated fatty liver disease. J Cachexia Sarcopenia Muscle 2023; 14(6): 2747-56.
[http://dx.doi.org/10.1002/jcsm.13351] [PMID: 37881112]

[25]   Alameri HF, Sanai FM, Al Dukhayil M, *et al.* Six Minute Walk Test to assess functional capacity in chronic liver disease patients. World J Gastroenterol 2007; 13(29): 3996-4001.
[http://dx.doi.org/10.3748/wjg.v13.i29.3996] [PMID: 17663517]

[26]   DeFronzo RA, Gunnarsson R, Björkman O, Olsson M, Wahren J. Effects of insulin on peripheral and splanchnic glucose metabolism in noninsulin-dependent (type II) diabetes mellitus. J Clin Invest 1985; 76(1): 149-55.

[http://dx.doi.org/10.1172/JCI111938] [PMID: 3894418]

[27]   Eguchi K, Manabe I, Oishi-Tanaka Y, *et al*. Saturated fatty acid and TLR signaling link β cell dysfunction and islet inflammation. Cell Metab 2012; 15(4): 518-33.
[http://dx.doi.org/10.1016/j.cmet.2012.01.023] [PMID: 22465073]

[28]   Gumucio JP, Qasawa AH, Ferrara PJ, *et al*. Reduced mitochondrial lipid oxidation leads to fat accumulation in myosteatosis. FASEB J 2019; 33(7): 7863-81.
[http://dx.doi.org/10.1096/fj.201802457RR] [PMID: 30939247]

[29]   Joost HG, Thorens B. The extended GLUT-family of sugar/polyol transport facilitators: nomenclature, sequence characteristics, and potential function of its novel members. Mol Membr Biol 2001; 18(4): 247-56.
[http://dx.doi.org/10.1080/09687680110090456] [PMID: 11780753]

[30]   Shoelson SE, Lee J, Goldfine AB. Inflammation and insulin resistance. J Clin Invest 2006; 116(7): 1793-801.
[http://dx.doi.org/10.1172/JCI29069] [PMID: 16823477]

[31]   Miljkovic I, Cauley JA, Wang PY, *et al*. Abdominal myosteatosis is independently associated with hyperinsulinemia and insulin resistance among older men without diabetes. Obesity (Silver Spring) 2013; 21(10): 2118-25.
[http://dx.doi.org/10.1002/oby.20346] [PMID: 23408772]

[32]   Khan RS, Bril F, Cusi K, Newsome PN. Modulation of insulin resistance in nonalcoholic fatty liver disease. Hepatology 2019; 70(2): 711-24.
[http://dx.doi.org/10.1002/hep.30429] [PMID: 30556145]

[33]   Martín-Domínguez V, González-Casas R, Mendoza-Jiménez-Ridruejo J, García-Buey L, Moreno-Otero R. Pathogenesis, diagnosis and treatment of non-alcoholic fatty liver disease. Rev Esp Enferm Dig 2013; 105(7): 409-20.
[http://dx.doi.org/10.4321/S1130-01082013000700006] [PMID: 24206551]

[34]   Marra F, Svegliati-Baroni G. Lipotoxicity and the gut-liver axis in NASH pathogenesis. J Hepatol 2018; 68(2): 280-95.
[http://dx.doi.org/10.1016/j.jhep.2017.11.014] [PMID: 29154964]

[35]   Fehrenbach H, Weiskirchen R, Kasper M, Gressner AM. Up-regulated expression of the receptor for advanced glycation end products in cultured rat hepatic stellate cells during transdifferentiation to myofibroblasts. Hepatology 2001; 34(5): 943-52.
[http://dx.doi.org/10.1053/jhep.2001.28788] [PMID: 11679965]

[36]   Lee Y, Kim SU, Song K, *et al*. Sarcopenia is associated with significant liver fibrosis independently of obesity and insulin resistance in nonalcoholic fatty liver disease: Nationwide surveys (KNHANES 2008-2011). Hepatology 2016; 63(3): 776-86.
[http://dx.doi.org/10.1002/hep.28376] [PMID: 26638128]

[37]   Davuluri G, Krokowski D, Guan BJ, *et al*. Metabolic adaptation of skeletal muscle to hyperammonemia drives the beneficial effects of l-leucine in cirrhosis. J Hepatol 2016; 65(5): 929-37.
[http://dx.doi.org/10.1016/j.jhep.2016.06.004] [PMID: 27318325]

[38]   Holeček M. Branched-chain amino acid supplementation in treatment of liver cirrhosis: Updated views on how to attenuate their harmful effects on cataplerosis and ammonia formation. Nutrition 2017; 41: 80-5.
[http://dx.doi.org/10.1016/j.nut.2017.04.003] [PMID: 28760433]

[39]   Qiu J, Thapaliya S, Runkana A, *et al*. Hyperammonemia in cirrhosis induces transcriptional regulation of myostatin by an NF-κB–mediated mechanism. Proc Natl Acad Sci USA 2013; 110(45): 18162-7.
[http://dx.doi.org/10.1073/pnas.1317049110] [PMID: 24145431]

[40]   Nishikawa H, Enomoto H, Ishii A, *et al*. Elevated serum myostatin level is associated with worse survival in patients with liver cirrhosis. J Cachexia Sarcopenia Muscle 2017; 8(6): 915-25.

[http://dx.doi.org/10.1002/jcsm.12212] [PMID: 28627027]

[41] Eliades M, Spyrou E, Agrawal N, *et al.* Meta-analysis: vitamin D and non-alcoholic fatty liver disease. Aliment Pharmacol Ther 2013; 38(3): 246-54.
[http://dx.doi.org/10.1111/apt.12377] [PMID: 23786213]

[42] Wang X, Li W, Zhang Y, Yang Y, Qin G. Association between vitamin D and non-alcoholic fatty liver disease/non-alcoholic steatohepatitis: results from a meta-analysis. Int J Clin Exp Med 2015; 8(10): 17221-34.
[PMID: 26770315]

[43] Ding N, Yu RT, Subramaniam N, *et al.* A vitamin D receptor/SMAD genomic circuit gates hepatic fibrotic response. Cell 2013; 153(3): 601-13.
[http://dx.doi.org/10.1016/j.cell.2013.03.028] [PMID: 23622244]

[44] Dunlop TW, Väisänen S, Frank C, Molnár F, Sinkkonen L, Carlberg C. The human peroxisome proliferator-activated receptor delta gene is a primary target of 1alpha,25-dihydroxyvitamin D3 and its nuclear receptor. J Mol Biol 2005; 349(2): 248-60.
[http://dx.doi.org/10.1016/j.jmb.2005.03.060] [PMID: 15890193]

[45] Pang Q, Qu K, Liu C, Zhang JY, Liu SS. Sarcopenia and nonalcoholic fatty liver disease: New evidence for low vitamin D status contributing to the link. Hepatology 2016; 63(2): 675.
[http://dx.doi.org/10.1002/hep.28010] [PMID: 26206563]

[46] Mizuno T, Hosoyama T, Tomida M, *et al.* Influence of vitamin D on sarcopenia pathophysiology: A longitudinal study in humans and basic research in knockout mice. J Cachexia Sarcopenia Muscle 2022; 13(6): 2961-73.
[http://dx.doi.org/10.1002/jcsm.13102] [PMID: 36237134]

[47] Cani PD, Bibiloni R, Knauf C, *et al.* Changes in gut microbiota control metabolic endotoxemia-induced inflammation in high-fat diet-induced obesity and diabetes in mice. Diabetes 2008; 57(6): 1470-81.
[http://dx.doi.org/10.2337/db07-1403] [PMID: 18305141]

[48] Ono Y, Sakamoto K. Lipopolysaccharide inhibits myogenic differentiation of C2C12 myoblasts through the Toll-like receptor 4-nuclear factor-κB signaling pathway and myoblast-derived tumor necrosis factor-α. PLoS One 2017; 12(7): e0182040.
[http://dx.doi.org/10.1371/journal.pone.0182040] [PMID: 28742154]

[49] Ono Y, Maejima Y, Saito M, *et al.* TAK-242, a specific inhibitor of Toll-like receptor 4 signalling, prevents endotoxemia-induced skeletal muscle wasting in mice. Sci Rep 2020; 10(1): 694.
[http://dx.doi.org/10.1038/s41598-020-57714-3] [PMID: 31959927]

[50] Pedersen BK, Akerstrom TC, Nielsen AR, *et al.* Role of myokine in exercise and metabolism. J Appl Physiol (1985) 2007; 03(3):1093-8.

[51] McPherron AC, Lawler AM, Lee SJ. Regulation of skeletal muscle mass in mice by a new TGF-p superfamily member. Nature 1997; 387(6628): 83-90.
[http://dx.doi.org/10.1038/387083a0] [PMID: 9139826]

[52] Rodriguez J, Vernus B, Chelh I, *et al.* Myostatin and the skeletal muscle atrophy and hypertrophy signaling pathways. Cell Mol Life Sci 2014; 71(22): 4361-71.
[http://dx.doi.org/10.1007/s00018-014-1689-x] [PMID: 25080109]

[53] García PS, Cabbabe A, Kambadur R, Nicholas G, Csete M. Brief-reports: elevated myostatin levels in patients with liver disease: a potential contributor to skeletal muscle wasting. Anesth Analg 2010; 111(3): 707-9.
[http://dx.doi.org/10.1213/ANE.0b013e3181eac1c9] [PMID: 20686014]

[54] Merli M, Dasarathy S. Sarcopenia in non-alcoholic fatty liver disease: Targeting the real culprit? J Hepatol 2015; 63(2): 309-11.
[http://dx.doi.org/10.1016/j.jhep.2015.05.014] [PMID: 26022692]

[55] Delogu W, Caligiuri A, Provenzano A, *et al.* Myostatin regulates the fibrogenic phenotype of hepatic stellate cells *via* c-jun N-terminal kinase activation. Dig Liver Dis 2019; 51(10): 1400-8.
[http://dx.doi.org/10.1016/j.dld.2019.03.002] [PMID: 31005555]

[56] Boström P, Wu J, Jedrychowski MP, *et al.* A PGC1-α-dependent myokine that drives brown-fat-like development of white fat and thermogenesis. Nature 2012; 481(7382): 463-8.
[http://dx.doi.org/10.1038/nature10777] [PMID: 22237023]

[57] Metwally M, Bayoumi A, Romero-Gomez M, *et al.* A polymorphism in the Irisin-encoding gene (FNDC5) associates with hepatic steatosis by differential miRNA binding to the 3′UTR. J Hepatol 2019; 70(3): 494-500.
[http://dx.doi.org/10.1016/j.jhep.2018.10.021] [PMID: 30389552]

[58] Park MJ, Kim DI, Choi JH, Heo YR, Park SH. New role of irisin in hepatocytes: The protective effect of hepatic steatosis *in vitro*. Cell Signal 2015; 27(9): 1831-9.
[http://dx.doi.org/10.1016/j.cellsig.2015.04.010] [PMID: 25917316]

[59] Tang H, Yu R, Liu S, Huwatibieke B, Li Z, Zhang W. Irisin inhibits hepatic cholesterol synthesis *via* AMPK-SREBP2 signaling. EBioMedicine 2016; 6: 139-48.
[http://dx.doi.org/10.1016/j.ebiom.2016.02.041] [PMID: 27211556]

[60] Zhou B, Ling L, Zhang F, *et al.* Fibronectin type III domain-containing 5 attenuates liver fibrosis *via* inhibition of hepatic stellate cell activation. Cell Physiol Biochem 2018; 48(1): 227-36.
[http://dx.doi.org/10.1159/000491722] [PMID: 30007970]

[61] Sugimoto T, Nakamura T, Yokoyama S, Fujisato T, Konishi S, Hashimoto T. Investigation of brain function-related myokine secretion by using contractile 3D-engineered muscle. Int J Mol Sci 2022; 23(10): 5723.
[http://dx.doi.org/10.3390/ijms23105723] [PMID: 35628536]

[62] Muñoz-Cánoves P, Scheele C, Pedersen BK, Serrano AL. Interleukin-6 myokine signaling in skeletal muscle: a double-edged sword? FEBS J 2013; 280(17): 4131-48.
[http://dx.doi.org/10.1111/febs.12338] [PMID: 23663276]

[63] Goyale A, Jain A, Smith C, *et al.* Assessment of non-alcoholic fatty liver disease (NAFLD) severity with novel serum-based markers: A pilot study. PLoS One 2021; 16(11): e0260313.
[http://dx.doi.org/10.1371/journal.pone.0260313] [PMID: 34813621]

[64] Haddad F, Xaldivar F, Cooper DM, *et al.* IL-6-induced skeletal muscle atrophy. J Appl Physiol (1985) 2005; 98(3): 911-7.

[65] Mauer J, Chaurasia B, Goldau J, *et al.* Signaling by IL-6 promotes alternative activation of macrophages to limit endotoxemia and obesity-associated resistance to insulin. Nat Immunol 2014; 15(5): 423-30.
[http://dx.doi.org/10.1038/ni.2865] [PMID: 24681566]

[66] Petersen AMW, Pedersen BK. The anti-inflammatory effect of exercise. J Appl Physiol (1985) 2005; 98(4): 1154-62.

CHAPTER 3

Impact of Nutrition and Exercise on Carbohydrate Metabolism

Yutaka Matsunaga[1,*]

[1] *Faculty of Human Health, Kurume University, Kurume, Japan*

Abstract: People consume nutrients such as carbohydrates, fats, proteins, vitamins, and minerals in their diet. Among these, carbohydrates and fats are mainly used by the body as energy. Lipids are stored in the body mainly in the form of triglycerides, whereas carbohydrates are primarily stored in the liver and skeletal muscles in the form of glycogen. Compared to fat, glycogen can be stored in much smaller quantities in the body. Glycogen utilization has also been shown to increase during exercise. When glycogen is depleted, exercise performance is impaired. Glycogen is, therefore, a valuable source of energy, and much research has been conducted on how to store glycogen and how to enhance glycogen recovery after exercise. In addition, managing glucose and glycogen through proper nutrition and exercise training is very important not only for improving athletic performance but also for maintaining and improving health. Therefore, this chapter focuses on the impact of nutrition and exercise on carbohydrate metabolism.

Keywords: Glycogen, Glucose, Liver, Metabolism, Skeletal muscle.

INTRODUCTION

People consume nutrients such as carbohydrates, fats, proteins, vitamins, and minerals in their diet. Among these, carbohydrates and fats are mainly used as energy for the body. Ingested carbohydrates are broken down by digestive enzymes such as amylase and are absorbed primarily in the small intestine. Carbohydrates absorbed in the small intestine are transported throughout the body in the form of glucose. This glucose is used for ATP (adenosine triphosphate) production or stored as glycogen. Glycogen is stored mainly in the liver and skeletal muscle, and the amount is approximately estimated to be 100 g in the liver and 500 g in skeletal muscle, for a total of about 600 g [1, 2].

It has been shown that glucose utilization increases during exercise compared to resting conditions [3]. This increase is due to a greater reliance on the glycolytic

---

[*] **Corresponding author Yutaka Matsunaga:** Faculty of Human Health, Kurume University, Kurume, Japan; E-mail: matsunaga_yutaka@kurume-u.ac.jp

Hiroaki Eshima, Ikuru Miura, Yutaka Matsunaga & Yuki Tomiga (Eds.)

system for energy production. Carbohydrates provide 4 kcal of energy per gram, but the body can store only a few thousand calories. This is a small amount compared to the vast amount of energy stored in the body in the form of triglycerides. Glycogen is a particularly important energy source because of the limited amount that can be stored. Much research has focused on strategies for pre-exercise glycogen storage and post-exercise glycogen replacement. In addition, managing glucose and glycogen through proper nutrition and exercise training is critical not only for improving athletic performance but also for maintaining and improving health. Therefore, this chapter focuses on the impact of nutrition and exercise on carbohydrate metabolism.

EXERCISE AND GLYCOGEN DEPLETION

During exercise, carbohydrates and lipids are the main sources of energy. Lipids have 9 kcal of energy per gram, while carbohydrates have 4 kcal per gram. Lipids have a high energy density, which has the advantage that when energy is stored in the form of triglycerides, they are less likely to gain weight. However, it takes more effort than carbohydrates to metabolize lipids and use them as energy. Therefore, during exercise, which requires quick movements, more readily available carbohydrates are used. In previous studies, it has been reported that prolonged exercise decreases glycogen in skeletal muscle [4]. Skeletal muscle glycogen is also reduced by brief periods of high-intensity exercise, such as 30 seconds of all-out exercise [5].

The decrease in skeletal muscle glycogen content associated with exercise occurs in an exercise intensity-dependent manner [3, 6, 7]. For example, Van Loon *et al.* examined changes in the percentage of energy substrate utilization during 40, 55, and 75% maximal workload (Wmax) exercise in elite cyclists. The results showed that at rest, lipid oxidation and carbohydrate oxidation accounted for 56% and 44% of total energy expenditure, respectively, whereas at 40% Wmax, lipid oxidation and carbohydrate oxidation accounted for 55% and 45%, respectively. At 55% Wmax, lipid oxidation was 49% and carbohydrate oxidation was 51%, and when exercise intensity was increased to 75% Wmax, lipid oxidation was 24% and carbohydrate oxidation was 76% [3]. Romijn *et al.* similarly evaluated energy substrate utilization during exercise at 25, 65, and 85% VO2max and reported increased glucose oxidation with increasing exercise intensity [6]. These data indicate that glucose utilization increases with increasing exercise intensity. It has also been reported that glucose tissue uptake increases with increasing exercise intensity and that at 65 and 85% VO2max exercise, carbohydrate oxidation greatly exceeds glucose uptake [6]. In other words, glucose utilization in skeletal muscle increases with exercise, and glycogen is more likely to be depleted than glucose uptake. In fact, it has been reported that glycogen decreases significantly in competitions such as soccer, in which long periods of running and short periods of sprinting are repeated [8].

Effects of Muscle Glycogen Depletion

Glycogen can be stored in the body in much smaller quantities than fat. For example, Guezennec *et al.* reported that A man whose weight is near 70 kg has approximately 15 kg of fat as triglycerides in adipose tissue, representing about 140,000 kcal [9]. In humans, on the other hand, given that the majority of glycogen is stored in skeletal muscle (~500 g) and liver (~100 g) [1], the amount of carbohydrates in the body is only a few thousand kcal. Also, with exercise, glycogen stores decrease significantly.

So, what are the effects of reduced glycogen in skeletal muscle? In a previous study, Xirouchaki *et al.* examined the impact on exercise capacity in mice in which glycogen synthase was knocked out, specifically in skeletal muscle.

The results showed that exercise performance decreased when skeletal muscle glycogen levels were reduced [10]. There are several factors that contribute to reduced exercise performance when skeletal muscle glycogen levels decrease, but they are not yet fully understood. One possibility is that reduced glycogen levels affect ATP resynthesis in the glycolytic system, which would be a limiting factor in exercise, especially during high-intensity exercise. In addition, glycogen is involved in Na^+, K^+, and ATPase activity [11], and reduced skeletal muscle glycogen is involved in Ca^{2+} release from the sarcoplasmic reticulum [12]. Furthermore, it has been reported that reduced Ca^{2+} release leads to reduced muscle tensile strength [13]. Thus, a decrease in skeletal muscle glycogen content may inhibit muscle contraction.

Effects of Liver Glycogen Depletion

The main storage tissues for glycogen are the liver and skeletal muscles, with the liver holding 100 g and skeletal muscles holding 500 g, for a total of about 600 g [1, 2]. Therefore, the liver, like skeletal muscles, stores a large amount of glycogen. The glycogen in skeletal muscles is broken down to produce ATP, which can then be used to contract muscles. On the other hand, the primary role of glycogen in the liver is to supply glucose to extrahepatic tissues and maintain blood glucose levels [14]. When blood glucose levels decrease, the liver acts as a glucose sensor, degrading glycogen and supplying glucose to the blood. The ability of the liver glycogen to maintain blood glucose levels for some time without causing immediate hypoglycemia during fasting is due to the function of liver glycogen. However, liver glycogen stores are also limited. Exercise raises the degradation of liver glycogen [15]. Wahren *et al.* reported that splanchnic glucose production increased progressively during exercise, reaching levels 3 to 5-fold above resting values at heavy workloads [16]. Ahlborg *et al.* also examined substrate utilization during 4 hours of exercise at 30% VO2max. They reported that glucose release from the liver increased during prolonged exercise and that blood glucose levels were maintained for 40 minutes after the start of exercise but then dropped to 70% of baseline levels as exercise continued. Total splanchnic glucose release was estimated at 75 g in 4 h, enough to deplete approximately 75% of liver glycogen stores [17]. When prolonged exercise decreases liver glycogen and glycogenesis cannot adequately compensate, liver glucose production decreases, and muscle glucose uptake can be limited by hypoglycemia [18]. Therefore, liver glycogen stores are related to exercise performance as well as skeletal muscle glycogen levels [19].

METHOD TO REDUCE GLYCOGEN DEPLETION

Carbohydrate Loading

Glycogen depletion decreases exercise performance. So, what can be done to prevent glycogen depletion? One way is nutritional intake. Glycogen levels are also affected by nutritional status. Bergström *et al.* measured skeletal muscle glycogen levels after three days of consumption of three diets with different carbohydrate contents: a mixed diet, a protein+fat diet (protein 1500 kcal + fat 1300 kcal), and a predominantly carbohydrate diet (carbohydrate 2300 kcal + protein 500 kcal) [20]. The results show that skeletal muscle glycogen concentration increased with increasing carbohydrate intake. Interestingly, when an exercise capacity test was conducted, the group that consumed a diet high in carbohydrates was able to sustain exercise longer. Thus, a technique called "carbohydrate loading" is used to increase glycogen stores through a diet high in carbohydrates [21].

Fat Adaptation

Carbohydrate loading was designed to increase the amount of glycogen stored in the body through diet and to increase the amount of carbohydrates available during exercise. Other methods include "fat adaptation ". Burke *et al.* examined the effects of consuming a high-carbohydrate diet or a high-fat diet of equal energy for 5 days in eight well-trained cyclists [22]. The results showed that the high-fat diet decreased RER during exercise. Muoio *et al.* also showed that a diet high in lipids improves lipid oxidation capacity and enhances exercise time to exhaustion [23]. Conversely, it has been reported that a diet high in lipids reduces performance [24, 25]. Although a diet high in lipids increases lipid utilization, further research may be needed to determine whether it is effective in improving performance.

Exercise Training

Glycogen utilization is influenced not only by nutritional status but also by exercise training. Research has shown that continuous endurance training leads to an increase in mitochondria, the cell organelles responsible for ATP production [26]. Additionally, it has been found that both high-intensity interval training (HIIT) and prolonged endurance exercises contribute to an increase in mitochondria, suggesting that there are methods to boost mitochondrial content in a shorter timeframe efficiently [27]. An increase in mitochondria enhances energy production through the oxidative system and reduces reliance on the glycolytic system for energy production during the same level of exercise. This shift in energy production means that more lipids are utilized for energy during exercise while the utilization of carbohydrates decreases. Improving mitochondrial density through exercise training can lead to more efficient energy utilization, favoring fat as a fuel over glycogen, which can have implications for endurance performance and overall energy management during physical activities.

GLYCOGEN RECOVERY AFTER EXERCISE

In the context of actual sporting competitions, it is common for athletes to undergo multiple exercise sessions within a single day, such as participating in qualifying rounds and finals or engaging in practice sessions in both the morning and afternoon. In these scenarios, the speed at which the body replenishes glycogen that was depleted during the first exercise session is believed to impact the outcome of the race and the effectiveness of the training. Previous research has indicated that improving glycogen recovery following exercise is associated with enhanced performance in subsequent exercise sessions [28, 29]. Below are some key points on how to enhance glycogen recovery (Fig. 1).

What to Ingest?

Glycogen synthesis is fundamentally the process through which glucose units are linked to form lengthy chains. Pascoe *et al.* demonstrated that following high-intensity weight resistance exercise, consuming either a 23% carbohydrate solution (1.5 g.kg-1) led to significant differences in glycogen recovery compared to a control group that ingested water [30]. After a 2-hour recovery period, there was no notable change in glycogen levels for the water group (from 101.3 ± 13.1 to 105.1 ± 13.1 mmol kg-1 wet weight). In contrast, the group that received carbohydrates exhibited a significant glycogen recovery (from 91.7 ± 11.8 to 117.6 ± 16.5 mmol kg-1 wet weight). Although glycogen recovery through glycogenesis in the liver has been reported to occur even during fasting after exercise [31], the amount of glycogen that can be replenished is minimal. Furthermore, it has been documented that there is a direct correlation between the quantity of carbohydrates consumed post-exercise and the glycogen stores thereafter [32]. Thus, it is crucial to consume carbohydrates, the essential building blocks of glycogen, to facilitate glycogen recovery.

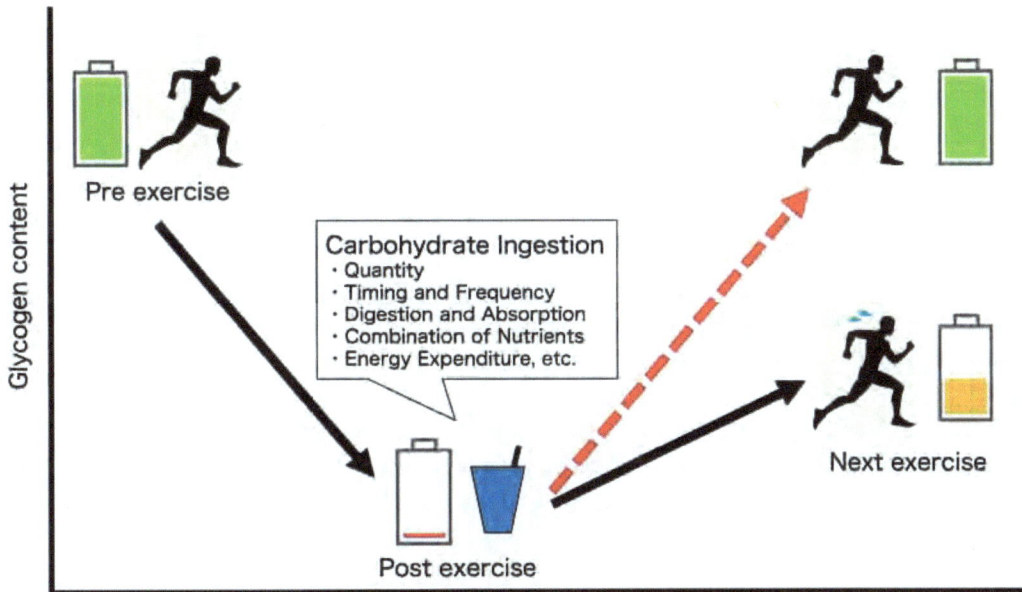

Fig. (1). Overview of methods to enhance glycogen recovery after exercise.

Regarding Quantity

The optimal amount of carbohydrate intake for enhancing glycogen recovery has been extensively studied. One study demonstrated that the rate of glycogen synthesis post-exercise was higher when 0.7 g.kg-1 of glucose was consumed compared to 0.35 g.kg-1 of carbohydrate [33]. Consuming 1.2 g of carbohydrates per kg of body weight per hour significantly improves muscle glycogen replenishment after exercise when compared to consuming lower amounts, such as 0.8 g per kg of body weight per hour [34]. However, no additional benefits in glycogen recovery are observed when carbohydrate intake increases from 1.5 g to 3.0 g per kg of body weight [35], suggesting there is a ceiling effect on the amount of carbohydrate that can be effectively used for glycogen resynthesis. Specifically, Jentjens and Jeukendrup have proposed that the optimal rate for glycogen synthesis is approximately 1.2 g per kg of body weight per hour [36]. This indicates a targeted range for carbohydrate consumption that optimizes glycogen recovery without exceeding what the body can efficiently utilize.

Timing and Frequency

Ivy *et al.* conducted a study focusing on the timing of carbohydrate intake after exercise [37]. They compared carbohydrate ingestion immediately after exercise ingestion with a 2-hour delay. They found that recovery 2 hours after ingestion was significantly higher in the group that ingested immediately after exercise (immediately after exercise ingestion: 7.7 mumol.g wet wt-1.h-1 v .s. 2 h postexercise ingestion: 2.5 mumol.g wet wt-1.h-1). Underlying these differences is the increased uptake of glucose after exercise. Previous studies have shown that high-intensity or prolonged endurance exercise results in a large decrease in skeletal muscle glycogen and a concomitant increase in glucose uptake [38]. The increase in glucose uptake after exercise lasts for about 30 minutes and returns to its original value 2 hours later [39]. Considering these factors, it is recommended that carbohydrates be consumed as soon as possible after the end of the exercise when skeletal muscle glucose uptake is high.

The frequency of carbohydrate intake has also been debated, with Burke *et al.* finding no difference in post-exercise glycogen stores over a 24-hour period when high-carbohydrate meals were consumed frequently as small snacks or as large meals [40]. During the short recovery time after exercise, it appears that frequent ingestion is associated with better glycogen recovery than large amounts [34]. There are also indications that small amounts of carbohydrates at frequent intervals may reduce the risk of gastrointestinal discomfort (*e.g.*, bloating) [36]. On the other hand, our group directly compared the effects of different feeding schedules on glycogen synthesis rates in laboratory animals [41]. The results showed that skeletal muscle glycogen recovered better in the Bolus group when 1.2 g/g BW of glucose was fed once immediately after exercise (Bolus) or divided into four doses of 0.3 mg/g Bw each (Pulse). This is expected to be due to the higher insulin secretion and increased blood glucose uptake in skeletal muscle when more sugar is ingested at one time. On the other hand, for the pulse group, skeletal muscle glycogen recovery was attenuated, whereas liver glycogen recovery was enhanced. The effect of different carbohydrate intake schedules on glycogen recovery may vary depending on the experimental conditions, and further investigation is needed.

Digestion and Absorption

Prior studies have reported that the rate of gastric emptying of glucose during exercise exceeds 1.5 g-min-1, while the maximum intestinal glucose absorption rate at rest is estimated to be ~1.3 g-min-1 [42]. In other words, glucose absorption is the rate-limiting step in nutrient supply, and enhancing digestion and absorption may affect glycogen recovery. Ingested carbohydrates are digested by digestive enzymes such as amylase and absorbed in the small intestine by Na+-coupled glucose cotransporters1 (SGLT1) and facilitative glucose transporter 2 (GLUT2) [43]. Kondo reported an increase in SGLT1 in the small intestine after 6 weeks of endurance training in laboratory animals [44]. This suggests that exercise training may affect digestion and absorption as well as skeletal muscle.

Other possibilities include the temperature of the ingested solution, which may affect digestive and absorptive function and subsequent peripheral tissue adaptation. Previous studies have shown that the gastric emptying rate increases in a temperature-dependent manner as the temperature of the ingested solution becomes colder [45]. It is possible that the coldness of the ingested solution increases the rate of gastric emptying, and the amount absorbed in the small intestine cannot keep up. In fact, in our study, we examined the effects of ingestion of three different carbohydrate solutions (4, 37, and 55°C) at various temperatures on glycogen recovery in animal experiments [46]. As a result, we reported that the warmer solution increased blood glucose concentration in the portal vein (an index of sugar absorption) and enhanced glycogen recovery in the liver.

Combination of Nutrients

While the recommended carbohydrate intake post-exercise is approximately [1, 2] g/kg of body weight (BW), consuming large amounts of carbohydrates at once may prove challenging. Consequently, research has explored the potential of augmenting carbohydrate intake with other nutrients to restore glycogen more efficiently. One notable strategy involves the combined intake of protein and carbohydrates. Studies have shown that the addition of protein or protein hydrolysate to carbohydrates post-exercise can boost glycogen recovery [34, 47, 48]. This effect is likely attributed to the synergistic action of these nutrients in enhancing insulin secretion and facilitating glucose uptake. Indeed, Morifuji discovered that the post-exercise consumption of carbohydrates and whey protein hydrolysate improves the phosphorylation of Akt, a key player in insulin signaling [49], thereby promoting glycogen replenishment. Moreover, the intake of a mix of proteins and carbohydrates has been shown to be beneficial not just for glycogen recovery in skeletal muscle but also for skeletal muscle protein synthesis [50]. However, it is important to note that there are also studies suggesting that carbohydrate plus protein intake does not enhance glycogen recovery [51]. Hall *et al.* observed this when carbohydrate intake was high (1.67 g/kg) and accompanied by whey protein hydrolysate (0.5 g/kg BW). It appears that when carbohydrate intake alone is sufficient to stimulate glycogen synthesis, the additional contribution of protein is minimal. Thus, while combining protein with carbohydrates may improve glycogen recovery efficiency with lesser amounts of carbohydrates and boost recovery efficiency, it might not necessarily increase the maximum quantity of glycogen that can be replenished.

Energy Expenditure

Energy expenditure is another critical factor influencing glycogen synthesis. Fushimi *et al.* demonstrated that the consumption of an acetic acid mixture following a period of fasting can enhance glycogen recovery in both the liver and skeletal muscle [52]. This effect is attributed to the activation of glycogenesis and the suppression of the glycolytic pathway. Conversely, some findings showthat consuming carbohydrates and casein hydrolysate during glycogen recovery post-exercise can increase energy expenditure and may actually hinder glycogen replenishment [53]. While there are relatively few studies directly examining the impact of energy substrate utilization on glycogen recovery, these findings suggest that the metabolic responses induced by different nutritional interventions can influence the efficiency of glycogen resynthesis. This underscores the importance of considering the metabolic context and energy demands when planning nutritional strategies for optimizing glycogen recovery after exercise.

METABOLIC DISEASE AND GLYCOGEN

Glucose absorbed by skeletal muscle can be utilized for ATP production, which is necessary for muscle contraction, or converted into glycogen. Research has highlighted that in diabetic patients, glucose uptake into skeletal muscle is diminished, leading to decreased rates of glycogen synthesis and reduced skeletal muscle glycogen stores [54, 55]. Given that skeletal muscle glycogen is a crucial energy source during exercise, its depletion can significantly restrict physical activity. Moreover, effective blood glucose management is essential for maintaining good health, necessitating enhanced glucose uptake and glycogen synthesis in skeletal muscle.

Exercise training has been reported to increase the quantity of GLUT4 protein, which plays a key role in glucose uptake [56], and enhance insulin sensitivity [57]. Consequently, exercise training has been associated with improved glycogen recovery [58, 59].

From a dietary perspective, the consumption of high glycemic index (GI) foods has been shown to be more beneficial for glycogen recovery post-exercise than low-GI foods, as they increase blood glucose concentration and insulin levels [60]. However, it is important to consider that in diabetic patients, postprandial hyperglycemia and the resultant insulin hypersecretion can elevate the risk of various metabolic diseases. One dietary modification could involve altering the types of carbohydrates consumed. For instance, Isomaltulose (palatinose), a naturally occurring disaccharide made of α-1,6-linked glucose and fructose [61], has been studied for its effects on blood glucose and insulin concentrations [62]. Consumption of Isomaltulose, as compared to sucrose, has been shown to cause lower increases in blood glucose and insulin levels. Koshinaka *et al.* [63] also reported that the intake of Isomaltulose, in contrast to starch, led to increased skeletal muscle glucose uptake and improved glycogen recovery post-exercise.

CONCLUDING REMARKS

This chapter has discussed the effects of nutritional intake and exercise on carbohydrate metabolism. Since glucose is the primary source of energy during exercise, many nutritional strategies have been used in sports settings. Managing glucose and glycogen through proper nutrition and exercise training is critical not only for improving athletic performance but also for maintaining and improving health.

REFERENCES

[1]   Jensen J, Rustad PI, Kolnes AJ, Lai YC. The role of skeletal muscle glycogen breakdown for regulation of insulin sensitivity by exercise. Front Physiol 2011; 2: 112.
[http://dx.doi.org/10.3389/fphys.2011.00112] [PMID: 22232606]

[2]   Murray B, Rosenbloom C. Fundamentals of glycogen metabolism for coaches and athletes. Nutr Rev 2018; 76(4): 243-59.
[http://dx.doi.org/10.1093/nutrit/nuy001] [PMID: 29444266]

[3]   Van Loon LJC, Greenhaff PL, Constantin-Teodosiu D, Saris WHM, Wagenmakers AJM. The effects of increasing exercise intensity on muscle fuel utilisation in humans. J Physiol 2001; 536(1): 295-304.
[http://dx.doi.org/10.1111/j.1469-7793.2001.00295.x] [PMID: 11579177]

[4]   Bergström J, Hultman E. A study of the glycogen metabolism during exercise in man. Scand J Clin Lab Invest 1967; 19(3): 218-28.
[http://dx.doi.org/10.3109/00365516709090629] [PMID: 6048626]

[5]   Gibala MJ, McGee SL, Garnham AP, Howlett KF, Snow RJ, Hargreaves M. Brief intense interval exercise activates AMPK and p38 MAPK signaling and increases the expression of PGC-1alpha in human skeletal muscle. J Appl Physiol (1985). 2009;106(3):929-934.

[6]   Romijn JA, Coyle EF, Sidossis LS, *et al.* Regulation of endogenous fat and carbohydrate metabolism in relation to exercise intensity and duration. Am J Physiol 1993; 265(3 Pt 1): E380-91.
[PMID: 8214047]

[7]   Chen ZP, Stephens TJ, Murthy S, *et al.* Effect of exercise intensity on skeletal muscle AMPK signaling in humans. Diabetes 2003; 52(9): 2205-12.
[http://dx.doi.org/10.2337/diabetes.52.9.2205] [PMID: 12941758]

[8]   Krustrup P, Mohr M, Steensberg A, Bencke J, Kjær M, Bangsbo J. Muscle and blood metabolites during a soccer game: implications for sprint performance. Med Sci Sports Exerc 2006; 38(6): 1165-74.
[http://dx.doi.org/10.1249/01.mss.0000222845.89262.cd] [PMID: 16775559]

[9]   Guezennec C. Role of lipids on endurance capacity in man. Int J Sports Med 1992; 13(S 1) (Suppl. 1): S114-8.
[http://dx.doi.org/10.1055/s-2007-1024612] [PMID: 1483746]

[10] Xirouchaki CE, Mangiafico SP, Bate K, *et al.* Impaired glucose metabolism and exercise capacity with muscle-specific glycogen synthase 1 (gys1) deletion in adult mice. Mol Metab 2016; 5(3): 221-32.
[http://dx.doi.org/10.1016/j.molmet.2016.01.004] [PMID: 26977394]

[11] Jensen R, Nielsen J, Ørtenblad N. Inhibition of glycogenolysis prolongs action potential repriming period and impairs muscle function in rat skeletal muscle. J Physiol 2020; 598(4): 789-803.
[http://dx.doi.org/10.1113/JP278543] [PMID: 31823376]

[12] Ørtenblad N, Nielsen J, Saltin B, Holmberg HC. Role of glycogen availability in sarcoplasmic reticulum Ca $^{2+}$ kinetics in human skeletal muscle. J Physiol 2011; 589(3): 711-25.
[http://dx.doi.org/10.1113/jphysiol.2010.195982] [PMID: 21135051]

[13] Olsson K, Cheng AJ, Al-Ameri M, *et al.* Impaired sarcoplasmic reticulum Ca $^{2+}$ release is the major cause of fatigue-induced force loss in intact single fibres from human intercostal muscle. J Physiol 2020; 598(4): 773-87.
[http://dx.doi.org/10.1113/JP279090] [PMID: 31785106]

[14] Bollen M, Keppens S, Stalmans W. Specific features of glycogen metabolism in the liver. Biochem J 1998; 336(Pt 1)(Pt 1): 19-31.
[http://dx.doi.org/10.1042/bj3360019]

[15] Gonzalez JT, Fuchs CJ, Betts JA, Van Loon LJC. Liver glycogen metabolism during and after prolonged endurance-type exercise. Am J Physiol Endocrinol Metab 2016; 311(3): E543-53.
[http://dx.doi.org/10.1152/ajpendo.00232.2016] [PMID: 27436612]

[16] Wahren J, Felig P, Ahlborg G, Jorfeldt L. Glucose metabolism during leg exercise in man. J Clin Invest 1971; 50(12): 2715-25.
[http://dx.doi.org/10.1172/JCI106772] [PMID: 5129319]

[17] Ahlborg G, Felig P, Hagenfeldt L, Hendler R, Wahren J. Substrate turnover during prolonged exercise in man. Splanchnic and leg metabolism of glucose, free fatty acids, and amino acids. J Clin Invest 1974; 53(4): 1080-90.
[http://dx.doi.org/10.1172/JCI107645] [PMID: 4815076]

[18] Richter EA, Hargreaves M. Exercise, GLUT4, and skeletal muscle glucose uptake. Physiol Rev 2013; 93(3): 993-1017.
[http://dx.doi.org/10.1152/physrev.00038.2012] [PMID: 23899560]

[19] López-Soldado I, Guinovart JJ, Duran J. Increased liver glycogen levels enhance exercise capacity in mice. J Biol Chem 2021; 297(2): 100976.
[http://dx.doi.org/10.1016/j.jbc.2021.100976] [PMID: 34284060]

[20] Bergström J, Hermansen L, Hultman E, Saltin B. Diet, muscle glycogen and physical performance. Acta Physiol Scand 1967; 71(2-3): 140-50.
[http://dx.doi.org/10.1111/j.1748-1716.1967.tb03720.x] [PMID: 5584523]

[21] Bussau V, Fairchild T, Rao A, Steele P, Fournier P. Carbohydrate loading in human muscle: an improved 1 day protocol. Eur J Appl Physiol 2002; 87(3): 290-5.
[http://dx.doi.org/10.1007/s00421-002-0621-5] [PMID: 12111292]

[22] Burke LM, Angus DJ, Cox GR, *et al.* Effect of fat adaptation and carbohydrate restoration on metabolism and performance during prolonged cycling. J Appl Physiol (1985) 2000; 89(6): 2413-21.

[23] Muoio DM, Leddy JJ, Horvath PJ, Aw AB, Pendergast DR. Effect of dietary fat on metabolic adjustments to maximal &OV0312;O2 and endurance in runners. Med Sci Sports Exerc 1994; 26(1): 81-8.
[http://dx.doi.org/10.1249/00005768-199401000-00014] [PMID: 8133743]

[24] Burke LM, Ross ML, Garvican-Lewis LA, *et al.* Low carbohydrate, high fat diet impairs exercise economy and negates the performance benefit from intensified training in elite race walkers. J Physiol 2017; 595(9): 2785-807.
[http://dx.doi.org/10.1113/JP273230] [PMID: 28012184]

[25]   Burke LM, Whitfield J, Heikura IA, *et al.* Adaptation to a low carbohydrate high fat diet is rapid but impairs endurance exercise metabolism and performance despite enhanced glycogen availability. J Physiol 2021; 599(3): 771-90.
[http://dx.doi.org/10.1113/JP280221] [PMID: 32697366]

[26]   Holloszy JO. Biochemical adaptations in muscle. Effects of exercise on mitochondrial oxygen uptake and respiratory enzyme activity in skeletal muscle. J Biol Chem 1967; 242(9): 2278-82.
[http://dx.doi.org/10.1016/S0021-9258(18)96046-1] [PMID: 4290225]

[27]   Little JP, Safdar A, Wilkin GP, Tarnopolsky MA, Gibala MJ. A practical model of low-volume high-intensity interval training induces mitochondrial biogenesis in human skeletal muscle: potential mechanisms. J Physiol 2010; 588(6): 1011-22.
[http://dx.doi.org/10.1113/jphysiol.2009.181743] [PMID: 20100740]

[28]   Alghannam AF, Jedrzejewski D, Tweddle MG, *et al.* Impact of muscle glycogen availability on the capacity for repeated exercise in man. Med Sci Sports Exerc 2016; 48(1): 123-31.
[http://dx.doi.org/10.1249/MSS.0000000000000737] [PMID: 26197030]

[29]   Casey A, Mann R, Banister K, *et al.* Effect of carbohydrate ingestion on glycogen resynthesis in human liver and skeletal muscle, measured by [13] C MRS. Am J Physiol Endocrinol Metab 2000; 278(1): E65-75.
[http://dx.doi.org/10.1152/ajpendo.2000.278.1.E65] [PMID: 10644538]

[30]   Pascoe DD, Costill DL, Fink WJ, Robergs RA, Zachwieja JJ. Glycogen resynthesis in skeletal muscle following resistive exercise. Med Sci Sports Exerc 1993; 25(3): 349-54.
[http://dx.doi.org/10.1249/00005768-199303000-00009] [PMID: 8455450]

[31]   Mæhlum S, Hermansen L. Muscle glycogen concentration during recovery after prolonged severe exercise in fasting subjects. Scand J Clin Lab Invest 1978; 38(6): 557-60.
[http://dx.doi.org/10.1080/00365517809108819] [PMID: 705238]

[32]   Burke LM, Kiens B, Ivy JL. Carbohydrates and fat for training and recovery. J Sports Sci 2004; 22(1): 15-30.
[http://dx.doi.org/10.1080/0264041031000140527] [PMID: 14971430]

[33]   Blom PC, Høstmark AT, Vaage O, Kardel KR, Maehlum S. Effect of different post-exercise sugar diets on the rate of muscle glycogen synthesis. Med Sci Sports Exerc 1987; 19(5): 491-6.
[http://dx.doi.org/10.1249/00005768-198710000-00012] [PMID: 3316904]

[34]   Van Loon LJC, Saris WHM, Kruijshoop M, Wagenmakers AJM. Maximizing postexercise muscle glycogen synthesis: carbohydrate supplementation and the application of amino acid or protein hydrolysate mixtures. Am J Clin Nutr 2000; 72(1): 106-11.
[http://dx.doi.org/10.1093/ajcn/72.1.106] [PMID: 10871568]

[35]   Ivy JL, Lee MC, Brozinick JT Jr, Reed MJ. Muscle glycogen storage after different amounts of carbohydrate ingestion. J Appl Physiol (1985). 1988;65(5):2018-2023.

[36]   Jentjens R, Jeukendrup AE. Determinants of post-exercise glycogen synthesis during short-term recovery. Sports Med 2003; 33(2): 117-44.
[http://dx.doi.org/10.2165/00007256-200333020-00004] [PMID: 12617691]

[37]   Ivy JL, Katz AL, Cutler CL, Sherman WM, Coyle EF. Muscle glycogen synthesis after exercise: effect of time of carbohydrate ingestion. J Appl Physiol (1985) 1988; 64(4): 1480-5.

[38]   Kawanaka K, Tabata I, Tanaka A, Higuchi M. Effects of high-intensity intermittent swimming on glucose transport in rat epitrochlearis muscle. J Appl Physiol (1985) 1998; 84(6): 1852-7.

[39]   Goodyear LJ, Hirshman MF, King PA, Horton ED, Thompson CM, Horton ES. Skeletal muscle plasma membrane glucose transport and glucose transporters after exercise. J Appl Physiol (1985) 1990; 68(1): 193-8.

[40]   Burke LM, Collier GR, Davis PG, Fricker PA, Sanigorski AJ, Hargreaves M. Muscle glycogen storage

after prolonged exercise: effect of the frequency of carbohydrate feedings. Am J Clin Nutr 1996; 64(1): 115-9.
[http://dx.doi.org/10.1093/ajcn/64.1.115] [PMID: 8669406]

[41]   Matsunaga Y, Takahashi K, Takahashi Y, Hatta H. Effects of glucose ingestion at different frequencies on glycogen recovery in mice during the early hours post exercise. J Int Soc Sports Nutr 2021; 18(1): 69.
[http://dx.doi.org/10.1186/s12970-021-00467-9] [PMID: 34743706]

[42]   Gonzalez J, Fuchs C, Betts J, Van Loon L. Glucose plus fructose ingestion for post-exercise recovery—greater than the sum of its parts? Nutrients 2017; 9(4): 344.
[http://dx.doi.org/10.3390/nu9040344] [PMID: 28358334]

[43]   Shirazi-Beechey SP. Molecular biology of intestinal glucose transport. Nutr Res Rev 1995; 8(1): 27-41.
[http://dx.doi.org/10.1079/NRR19950005] [PMID: 19094278]

[44]   Kondo S, Fukazawa A, Karasawa T, Terada S. Effects of long-term exercise training for different durations on pancreatic amylase activity and intestinal glucose transporter content in rats. Physiol Rep 2019; 7(20): e14255.
[http://dx.doi.org/10.14814/phy2.14255] [PMID: 31650713]

[45]   Costill DL, Saltin B. Factors limiting gastric emptying during rest and exercise. J Appl Physiol 1974; 37(5): 679-83.
[http://dx.doi.org/10.1152/jappl.1974.37.5.679] [PMID: 4436193]

[46]   Matsunaga Y, Koyama S, Takahashi K, *et al.* Effects of post-exercise glucose ingestion at different solution temperatures on glycogen repletion in mice. Physiol Rep 2021; 9(18): e15041.
[http://dx.doi.org/10.14814/phy2.15041] [PMID: 34553503]

[47]   Zawadzki KM, Yaspelkis BB 3rd, Ivy JL. Carbohydrate-protein complex increases the rate of muscle glycogen storage after exercise. J Appl Physiol (1985) 1992; 72(5): 1854-9.

[48]   Ivy JL, Goforth HW Jr, Damon BM, McCauley TR, Parsons EC, Price TB. Early postexercise muscle glycogen recovery is enhanced with a carbohydrate-protein supplement. J Appl Physiol (1985) 2002; 93(4): 1337-44.

[49]   Morifuji M, Kanda A, Koga J, Kawanaka K, Higuchi M. Post-exercise carbohydrate plus whey protein hydrolysates supplementation increases skeletal muscle glycogen level in rats. Amino Acids 2010; 38(4): 1109-15.
[http://dx.doi.org/10.1007/s00726-009-0321-0] [PMID: 19593593]

[50]   Howarth KR, Moreau NA, Phillips SM, Gibala MJ. Coingestion of protein with carbohydrate during recovery from endurance exercise stimulates skeletal muscle protein synthesis in humans. J Appl Physiol (1985) 2009; 106(4): 1394-402.

[51]   Van Hall G, Shirreffs SM, Calbet JA. Muscle glycogen resynthesis during recovery from cycle exercise: no effect of additional protein ingestion. J Appl Physiol (1985) 2000; 88(5): 1631-6.

[52]   Fushimi T, Tayama K, Fukaya M, *et al.* Acetic acid feeding enhances glycogen repletion in liver and skeletal muscle of rats. J Nutr 2001; 131(7): 1973-7.
[http://dx.doi.org/10.1093/jn/131.7.1973] [PMID: 11435516]

[53]   Matsunaga Y, Sakata Y, Yago T, Nakamura H, Shimizu T, Takeda Y. Effects of glucose with casein peptide supplementation on post-exercise muscle glycogen resynthesis in C57BL/6J mice. Nutrients 2018; 10(6): 753.
[http://dx.doi.org/10.3390/nu10060753] [PMID: 29891805]

[54]   Shulman GI, Rothman DL, Jue T, Stein P, DeFronzo RA, Shulman RG. Quantitation of muscle glycogen synthesis in normal subjects and subjects with non-insulin-dependent diabetes by 13C nuclear magnetic resonance spectroscopy. N Engl J Med 1990; 322(4): 223-8.
[http://dx.doi.org/10.1056/NEJM199001253220403] [PMID: 2403659]

[55]   He J, Kelley DE. Muscle glycogen content in type 2 diabetes mellitus. Am J Physiol Endocrinol Metab 2004; 287(5): E1002-7.
[http://dx.doi.org/10.1152/ajpendo.00015.2004] [PMID: 15251866]

[56]   Terada S, Yokozeki T, Kawanaka K, *et al.* Effects of high-intensity swimming training on GLUT-4 and glucose transport activity in rat skeletal muscle. J Appl Physiol (1985) 2001; 90(6): 2019-24.

[57]   Hayashi T, Wojtaszewski JF, Goodyear LJ. Exercise regulation of glucose transport in skeletal muscle. Am J Physiol 1997; 273(6): E1039-51.
[PMID: 9435517]

[58]   Ren JM, Semenkovich CF, Gulve EA, Gao J, Holloszy JO. Exercise induces rapid increases in GLUT4 expression, glucose transport capacity, and insulin-stimulated glycogen storage in muscle. J Biol Chem 1994; 269(20): 14396-401.
[http://dx.doi.org/10.1016/S0021-9258(17)36636-X] [PMID: 8182045]

[59]   Nakatani A, Han DH, Hansen PA, *et al.* Effect of endurance exercise training on muscle glycogen supercompensation in rats. J Appl Physiol (1985) 1997; 82(2): 711-5.

[60]   Burke LM, Collier GR, Hargreaves M. Muscle glycogen storage after prolonged exercise: effect of the glycemic index of carbohydrate feedings. J Appl Physiol (1985) 1993; 75(2): 1019-23.

[61]   Lina BAR, Jonker D, Kozianowski G. Isomaltulose (Palatinose®): a review of biological and toxicological studies. Food Chem Toxicol 2002; 40(10): 1375-81.
[http://dx.doi.org/10.1016/S0278-6915(02)00105-9] [PMID: 12387299]

[62]   Kawai K, Okuda Y, Yamashita K. Changes in blood glucose and insulin after an oral palatinose administration in normal subjects. Endocrinol Jpn 1985; 32(6): 933-6.
[http://dx.doi.org/10.1507/endocrj1954.32.933] [PMID: 3914416]

[63]   Koshinaka K, Ando R, Sato A. Short-term replacement of starch with isomaltulose enhances both insulin-dependent and -independent glucose uptake in rat skeletal muscle. J Clin Biochem Nutr 2018; 63(2): 113-22.
[http://dx.doi.org/10.3164/jcbn.17-98] [PMID: 30279622]

CHAPTER 4

Brain Health in Metabolic Disease and Exercise

Yuki Tomiga[1,*]

[1] *Faculty of Sports and Health Science, Fukuoka University, Fukuoka, Japan*

Abstract: Modern lifestyles, such as a Western diet, excessive food consumption, and physical inactivity, are closely associated with brain health and noncommunicable diseases, including type 2 diabetes. Epidemiological evidence suggests that an unhealthy lifestyle leads to impaired brain health, manifesting in conditions such as depression and anxiety. Conversely, mental illness can contribute to the development of type 2 diabetes. Thus, it has been suggested that there is a bidirectional relationship between brain health and metabolic diseases, but the detailed mechanisms remain unclear.

Exercise is considered the primary choice for the treatment of obesity or type 2 diabetes. This is attributed to the fact that increased physical activity contributes to a reduction in body weight and the accumulation of excess adipose tissue. Furthermore, it has long been recognized that exercise enhances brain health. Recent studies have revealed that, in addition to these indirect effects, exercise exerts its beneficial effects by releasing bioactive substances. This chapter presents how metabolic diseases affect brain health and how exercise mitigates these detrimental effects, focusing particularly on the molecular mechanisms in the brain.

Keywords: Anxiety, Brain, Cognitive function, Diabetes, Depression, Hippocampus, Obesity.

INTRODUCTION

Obesity is defined as an excess of body adiposity. According to a report from the World Health Organization, worldwide obesity has nearly tripled since 1975, and 39% of adults aged 18 years and over were overweight in 2016, and 13% were obese. From this situation, in 2023, WHO advocated the *WHO acceleration plan to stop obesity* [1]. Overweight and obesity are central to the risk of metabolic syndrome, predisposing individuals to insulin resistance, hypertension, and dyslipidemia, all of which are risk factors for metabolic syndrome [2], and then progresses to the pathology of type 2 diabetes. Epidemiological research suggests that depression rates are twice as high among persons with diabetes as among

---

[*] **Corresponding author Yuki Tomiga:** Faculty of Sports and Health Science, Fukuoka University, Fukuoka, Japan; E-mail: tomiga0507@gmail.com

Hiroaki Eshima, Ikuru Miura, Yutaka Matsunaga & Yuki Tomiga (Eds.)

persons without diabetes [3]. In addition, diabetes is associated with an increased risk of psychological disturbance, especially for those with more diabetes-related complications [4]. Based on these studies, it has been considered as evidence that diabetes (and its complications) increases the risk of mental disorders. The causal relationship between metabolic and mental disorders remained unclear, but accumulating evidence suggested that it might appear to be bidirectional [5]. It is well known that physical activity, such as regular exercise, is beneficial for our health. It remained unclear whether the effect was simply due to the improvement of obesity or the effect of exercise itself. Very recent studies have revealed that exercise has its effects on the whole body, including the brain, through diverse mechanisms.

This chapter outlines the negative effects of metabolic diseases on brain health, especially in depression and anxiety, and the beneficial effects of exercise in improving them.

IMPAIRED BRAIN HEALTH IN METABOLIC DISEASE

With the recent westernization of diets, obesity has been increasing on a global scale and is already well-known to be a risk factor for various diseases [6]. In the 1980s, the ideal body weight approach was replaced by BMI, and the commonly used cutoffs for overweight (BMI 25–30) and obesity (BMI >30), for both men and women, were adopted to define obesity in adults [7]. Excess energy due to excessive lipid intake leads to obesity and the associated skeletal muscle insulin resistance and impaired glucose tolerance, which are major factors in type 2 diabetes mellitus. Although previous studies on obesity and glucose metabolism have focused on adipocytes [8 - 10] and skeletal muscle [11 - 13], recent studies have revealed that obesity also has important effects on brain function. For example, epidemiological studies reported that Western eating habits and being overweight are associated with reduced hippocampal volume [14, 15]. Western eating habits have also been found to be associated with psychiatric disorders such as depression and anxiety [16]. Insulin resistance is a prediabetic stage. A systematic review revealed a small but significant cross-sectional association between depression and insulin resistance [17]. In a study that investigated the association between metabolic syndrome and mood disorders, metabolic syndrome is associated with depressive symptoms but not anxiety in both men and women, irrespective of overweight/obesity status [18]. Further, patients with diabetes with both minor and major depression are associated with increased mortality [19].

Meanwhile, evidence suggests that a bidirectional relationship, in other words, mental illness, increases the risk of type 2 diabetes [5]. Eaton *et al.* reported in the

90s that major depressive disorder signals an increased risk for the onset of type 2 diabetes [20]. Also, individuals with newly diagnosed diabetes were 30% more likely to have had a previous history of depression compared with people without diabetes [21]. Interestingly, this relationship between mental illness and metabolic dysfunctions is observed not only in adulthood. According to Shomaker *et al.*, children's depressive symptoms were a significant predictor of follow-up HOMA-IR, fasting insulin, and fasting glucose levels [22]. A more recent study reported that persistently high fasting insulin levels from age 9 years were associated with psychosis at 24 years, and puberty-onset body mass index increase was associated with depression at 24 years [23].

In summary, obesity and overweight and the resulting metabolic disorders and psychiatric disorders, including depression, are bidirectional. Furthermore, childhood depression (or metabolic parameters such as high insulin levels) may be a predictor of future metabolic parameters (or depressive symptoms).

IMPAIRED NEUROGENESIS AND MOLECULAR MECHANISMS IN THE BRAIN IN METABOLIC DISEASE

Metabolic disorders are associated with impairment of brain health; however, these regulating mechanisms are not fully understood. In this section, we focus on mature hippocampal neurogenesis and molecular signaling within the hippocampus as the underlying mechanisms. As the hippocampus is a site of structural and functional pathology in most psychiatric disorders, it plays a crucial role in their manifestation. Therefore, a hippocampal-based treatment approach has been proposed to combat the cognitive deficits and mood dysregulation that are hallmarks of psychiatric disorders [24]. Adult hippocampal neurogenesis, the generation of new neurons in the adult dentate gyrus (DG), is an important event for the maintenance or regulation of brain function. Adult hippocampal neurogenesis is first discovered by Joseph Altman in 1963 [25]. In animal studies, mice lacking adult neurogenesis increased response to stress, which elevated blood glucocorticoid corticosterone [26]. Chronic high corticosterone reduces adult hippocampal neurogenesis in both males and females [27]. In addition, the above-mentioned adult neurogenesis-deficient mice also showed increased anxiety and depression-like behaviors [26]. In contrast, antidepressant treatment increased adult hippocampal neurogenesis [28, 29] and reduced depressive behaviors [30].

Brain-derived neurotrophic factor (BDNF) is a member of the neurotrophic family of proteins and is one of the key factors that affect cognitive functions and mental illness. BDNF is expressed in the central nervous system and is highly in the limbic area, which is important for effective regulation. BDNF regulates the development, survival, and differentiation of neurons through its high-affinity receptor, tropomyosin-related kinase B (TrkB corded by *Trkb* gene). Rodent study demonstrates that acute stress downregulates hippocampal BDNF messenger RNA expression [31]. *Trkb* is required for cell proliferation and adult hippocampal neurogenesis [32].

In rodent metabolic disease models, dietary models using high-fat diet (HFD) and genetically type 2 diabetic models are widely used. Although there is some discrepancy between models, in general, HFD and *db/db* mice have impaired cognitive functions such as spatial memory function and mood behavior [33 - 35]. In *db/db* mice, hippocampal BDNF expression levels are blunted [35, 36] and accompanied by decreased dendritic spine density in the DG [36]. In a study using a dietary obese mouse model induced by HFD, HFD significantly decreased the numbers of newly generated cells in the dentate gyrus of the hippocampus without neuronal loss, decreased the levels of hippocampal BDNF [37 - 39], and increased inflammatory responses in the hippocampus [40, 41]. In addition, HFD causes sex-specific deficits in adult hippocampal neurogenesis [42]. The genetic mouse model of obesity and diabetes has chronically elevated adrenal steroid hormones, such as glucocorticoids. Pharmacological inhibition of adrenal steroidogenesis attenuates structural and functional impairments by regulating plasticity among dendritic spines in the hippocampus of *db/db* mice [43]. Fourrier *et al.* reported that chronic inflammation in the hippocampus leads to anxiety-like behaviors [44]. In particular, tumor necrosis factor (TNF) -α, which is an inflammatory cytokine, is associated with behavioral abnormalities in *db/db* mice [44]. In summary, it is considered that HFD or obesity induces systemic and hippocampal inflammation and subsequently reduces hippocampal BDNF and cognitive deficit.

Another system that is linked to several neuronal and behavioral processes is the nitrergic system. Nitric oxide (NO) is a signaling molecule that is ubiquitously expressed throughout the body. NO regulates multiple biological processes and functions as a neuronal messenger in the brain. NO is synthesized from its precursor L-arginine by three isoforms of NO synthase (NOS), designated neuronal NOS (nNOS), inducible NOS (iNOS), and endothelial NOS (eNOS). In the adult brain, the major form of NOS in the central nervous system is nNOS [45]. Abbot and Nahm proposed potential concentration-dependent effects of NO [46]. NO appears to exert neuroprotective effects at low to moderate concentrations, whereas NO becomes neurotoxic as the concentration increases, and excessive NO production can cause oxidative stress to neurons, ultimately impairing neuronal function and resulting in neuronal cell death [46]. Indeed, in the case of Alzheimer's disease (AD), which is a progressive neurodegenerative disorder, aberrant expression of nNOS in those neurons that are particularly vulnerable in AD and transcriptional induction of nNOS might be an early event in the process of neurodegeneration [47]. In animal models, chronic mild stress increased depression-like behaviors accompanied by selectively up-regulated nNOS expression in the adult hippocampus [48]. In contrast, selective nNOS inhibition reversed stress-induced impairment of neurogenesis [48] and exerted antidepressant and anxiolytic properties [48 - 50]. Interestingly, similar to stress, HFD also increases hippocampal nNOS and is associated with anxiety-like behaviors [51, 52]. HFD-induced excess hippocampal nNOS expression appears to occur in a relatively later period of HFD consumption (7-12 weeks) but not in the early period (2 weeks) [51].

These findings suggest that psychiatric disorders such as depression and anxiety, which are said to be associated with HFD and Western diets, may result from impaired brain function in the brain (especially the hippocampus).

EXERCISE IN BRAIN HEALTH

Aristotle, who was a peripatetic philosopher, thought and discussed walking with his students. In such a way, since ancient times, it has been known that moderate physical activity may enhance brain function. This fact is one of the oldest evidence for a relationship between exercise and brain function. In recent years, in support of this, there have been accumulated findings that exercise affects brain health, including cognitive function, mood, learning, and memory.

Nowadays, it is well known that regular physical activity can significantly improve cognitive function and mental health and lessen symptoms of depression, anxiety, and stress [53, 54]. In a randomized controlled trial with 120 older adults, Ericson *et al.* showed that aerobic exercise training increases the size of the anterior hippocampus, leading to improvements in spatial memory [55]. Exercise training increased hippocampal volume by 2%, effectively reversing age-related loss in volume by 1 to 2 years. Also, they demonstrate that increased hippocampal volume is associated with greater serum levels of BDNF, a mediator of neurogenesis in the dentate gyrus [55]. Not only regular chronic exercise but much research has been performed to understand how a single bout of exercise (also referred to as acute exercise) affects cognitive performance [56]. It was reported that submaximal aerobic exercise performed for periods up to 60 min facilitates specific aspects of information processing; however, extended exercise that leads to dehydration compromises both information processing and memory functions [57]. Also, 30 min of moderate-intensity treadmill exercise improves the mood and well-being of patients with major depressive disorders [58]. Acute exercise-related cognitive performance improvement is characterized by a reduction in reaction time. A very recent study revealed that acute supine cycling exercise released endogenous dopamine (DA) and that this release was correlated with improved reaction time [59]. In a study examining the effects of exercise therapy and pharmacological treatment for major depression, after 4 months, patients in both groups exhibited significant improvement. After 10 months, however, remitted subjects in the exercise group had significantly lower relapse rates than subjects in the medication group [60]. Thus, unlike pharmacological treatments, the effects of exercise training on mood regulation have been shown to persist long after exercise is stopped potentially.

In summary, this evidence indicates that not only regular exercise intervention but even a single exercise session can have beneficial effects on brain function, and furthermore, these effects may be maintained for a certain period after exercise intervention is discontinued.

EFFECTS OF MOLECULAR MECHANISMS OF EXERCISE ON COGNITIVE FUNCTIONS AND METABOLIC DISORDERS-RELATED BRAIN DYSFUNCTION

Firstly, Neeper *et al.* reported that physical activity, such as exercise, increases BDNF in the murine brain [61]. Hippocampal and cerebral cortical BDNFs were increased by exercise with a running wheel for 2, 4, and 7 nights [61]. Since inhibiting BDNF action blocks the benefit of exercise on cognitive function, hippocampal BDNF mediates the efficacy of exercise on synaptic plasticity and cognition. There are some age-related differences in BDNF protein expression by exercise training in the hippocampus [62]. After 7 days of exercise, hippocampal BDNF protein levels were increased in young (2 months), late middle-aged (15 months), and old (24 months) mice, but after 28 days, these effects disappeared [63]. Also, there was a significant difference in the quantity of BDNF protein between sexes [64]. Chronic mild stress decreased the quantity of BDNF protein and sucrose preference, which is an indicator of depressive-like behaviors in female mice compared to male mice [64]. In a meta-analysis of 9 studies, exercise training effects on BDNF levels were greater in studies utilizing female rodents compared to studies on male rodents [65, 66]. Another study reported a relationship between hippocampal BDNF and nNOS in running exercise, accompanied by hippocampal region specificity [67]. BDNF protein levels in the hippocampus were increased in both the dorsal and ventral regions, but nNOS protein levels were only decreased in the ventral region, which contributes to mood behaviors [67]. These studies revealed that running exercise training decreased hippocampal nNOS [67], suggesting that exercise mediates similar signaling pathways with anti-depressants, as reported by Zhang *et al.* [50]. In addition, gene expression of these molecules is regulated by the changes in DNA methylation, which is one of the epigenetic modifications [67, 68]. Epigenetics is defined as the mechanisms regulating gene expression independent of DNA sequence, and epigenetic patterns are known to be inherited by the next generation of cells after cell division. Thus, it has been suggested that the mechanism by which the effects of exercise are maintained over time may involve epigenetic changes within the central nervous system.

In addition, as mentioned above, hippocampal BDNF levels decreased in HFD and type 2 diabetic animal models BDNF [36, 38]. These metabolic disorder-related negative changes were reversed by running exercise training. Voluntary running and caloric restriction exert additive effects on hippocampal BDNF levels in wild-type mice. The *db/db* mice also respond to running and caloric restriction but with smaller increases in hippocampal BDNF concentrations [36]. Cai *et al.* reported that dietary obesity can induce hippocampal endoplasmic reticulum stress (ERS) in male SD rats, and excessive hippocampal ERS plays a critical role in decreasing the levels of BDNF and synaptic protein synaptophysin (SYN). Moreover, aerobic exercise can activate hippocampal Nrf2 and HO-1, which play a role in anti-ERS, anti-inflammation, and anti-apoptosis in peripheral tissues, to relieve ERS and heighten BDNF and SYN production in obese rats [69]. Meanwhile, the Otsuka Long–Evans Tokushima fatty (OLETF) rat is also known as a useful type 2 diabetic model. Exercise training rescued cognitive dysfunction, such as impaired spatial memory in OLETF rats, but hippocampal BDNF levels were not recovered by exercise [70]. In obesity or type 2 diabetes, a metabolic abnormal state increases nNOS protein levels in the hippocampus [51, 52]. Shortening, which is a trans fatty acid widely used in fast food, also induced hippocampal nNOS, and selective nNOS inhibition recovered shortening-induced depressive-like behaviors [71]. Tomiga *et al.* showed that exercise training rescued HFD-induced excess hippocampal nNOS expression as untread control levels [52]. Interestingly, there were no significant effects of exercise within one week that did not alter HFD-induced hippocampal nNOS expression, but within six weeks, HFD-related alterations decreased [51]. Collectively, HFD and obesity lead to cognitive dysfunctions such as depressive and anxiety effects and impaired spatial memory function due to decreased BDNF in the hippocampus and enhanced nitric oxide signaling. However, in many cases, these effects can be reversed by exercise.

ROLE OF ORGAN CROSSTALK IN EXERCISE IN METABOLIC DISORDERS AND BRAIN HEALTH

Regular exercise has beneficial effects for multiple organs, prescribing exercise as medicine in the treatment of 26 different diseases: psychiatric diseases (depression, anxiety, stress, schizophrenia); neurological diseases (dementia, Parkinson's disease, multiple sclerosis); metabolic diseases (obesity, hyperlipidemia, metabolic syndrome, polycystic ovarian syndrome, type 2 diabetes, type 1 diabetes); cardiovascular diseases (hypertension, coronary heart disease, heart failure, cerebral apoplexy, and claudication intermittent); pulmonary diseases (chronic obstructive pulmonary disease, asthma, cystic fibrosis); musculo-skeletal disorders (osteoarthritis, osteoporosis, back pain, rheumatoid arthritis); and cancer [72]. Recent research has revealed that these diverse effects of exercise may be due to crosstalk between organs, for example, skeletal muscle to brain.

Today, it is well known that skeletal muscle is an endocrine organ that releases certain hormones, and the bioactive substances derived from skeletal muscle that are released from skeletal muscle are called "myokine". Exercise, in other words, skeletal muscle contraction, is one trigger that induces and releases myokine expression in skeletal muscle.

It is well known that exercise stimulates peroxisome proliferator-activated receptor gamma coactivator 1-alpha (PGC-1α), which is a key regulator for mitochondria biogenesis in skeletal muscle [73]. PGC1-α expression in muscle stimulates an increase in expression of fibronectin-domain III containing 5 (FNDC5), a membrane protein that is cleaved and secreted as an exercise-induced myokine, irisin, which is named after Iris, the Greek goddess of rainbows [74]. After this breakthrough, many studies have reported that irisin acts as a beneficial exercise messenger for multiple organs, including the brain.

A single bout of exercise increased blood irisin levels in humans and mice [75, 76]. FNDC5, which is the precursor of irisin, is increased by DG after exercise, accompanied by increased neurogenesis and reduced depressive-like behaviors [77, 78]. Exercise stimulates increased hippocampal *Fndc5* gene expression through a PGC-1α pathway [79]. This elevated *Fndc5* gene expression, in turn, stimulated*Bdnf* gene expression [79]. Islam *et al.* revealed that global FNDC knock-out (KO) mice impaired exercise-related cognitive dysfunction [80]. Irisin is a crucial regulator of the cognitive benefits of exercise and is a potential therapeutic agent for treating cognitive disorders, including AD [80]. Another study has found that cathepsin B (CTSB) is a novel myokine that is important for the cognitive and neurogenic benefits of running exercise [81]. *In vivo* analysis, recombinant CTSB treatment increased doublecortin and BDNF in neural progenitor cells [81]. In humans, 4 months of treadmill exercise training increased CTSB in blood, and there was a positive correlation between memory function and changes in CTSB level after 4 months of treadmill exercise [81]. Lactate is released into the blood after exercise from skeletal muscle and is recognized as one of the myokines. The metabolite lactate crosses the blood-brain barrier and induces Bdnf expression and TRKB signaling in the hippocampus [82]. Lactate-dependent increases in BDNF were associated with improved spatial learning and memory retention [82]. Thus, the knowledge that myokine released from skeletal muscle by exercise improves brain function is accumulating.

Another possible mechanism is an exercise-induced adipose tissue-derived cytokine called "adipokine". Subcutaneous white adipose tissue (scWAT) is intrinsically different from visceral white adipose tissue (vWAT) and produces substances that can act systemically to improve glucose metabolism [83]. Surprisingly, intraperitoneal implantation of exercise-trained scWAT into the abdominal cavity of recipient mice improved HFD-induced glucose tolerance as exercise did [84]. In addition, Takahashi *et al.* identified a novel exercise-induced adipokine, transforming growth factor (TGF)-β2 [85]. TGF-β2 treatment improved glucose intolerance and reduced serum-free fatty acid in obese mice[85]. They found that TGF-β2 is induced by lactate signaling [85]. Although there is no direct evidence so far, it is possible that unknown exercise-induced adipokines may be involved in the regulation of brain function during exercise *via* crosstalk between adipose tissue and the brain (Fig. **1**).

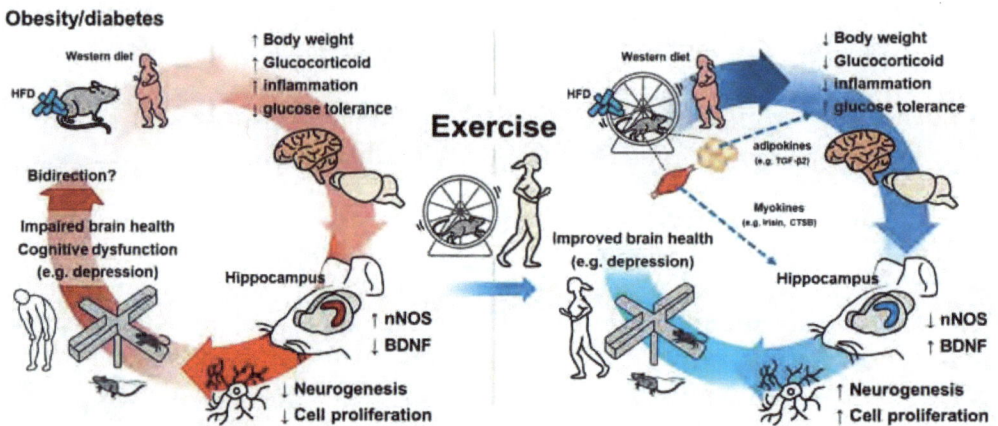

Fig. (1). Schematic illustration of metabolic disorders-related brain dysfunction and effects of exercise.

CONCLUDING REMARKS

This chapter discussed the effects of metabolic disorders, such as obesity and type 2 diabetes, on brain health, as well as the ameliorative effects of exercise. It is well known that exercise enhances brain function, and it is becoming clear that exercise improves brain function in metabolic disorders. However, much remains unclear regarding how exercise exerts its effects. Recent evidence suggests that the systemic effects of exercise appear to be more complex and regulated through multiorgan linkages. Challenges in elucidating these mechanisms have the potential to construct new therapeutic strategies that will lead to the maintenance and promotion of brain health.

REFERENCES

[1]   WHO. The WHO Acceleration Plan to STOP Obesity: progress from WHA 75 Nutrition and Food Safety Department, WHO HQ. 2023; https://www.who.int/publications/i/item/9789240075634

[2]   O'Neill S, O'Driscoll L. Metabolic syndrome: a closer look at the growing epidemic and its associated pathologies. Obes Rev 2015; 16(1): 1-12.
[http://dx.doi.org/10.1111/obr.12229] [PMID: 25407540]

[3]   Anderson RJ, Freedland KE, Clouse RE, Lustman PJ. The prevalence of comorbid depression in adults with diabetes: a meta-analysis. Diabetes Care 2001; 24(6): 1069-78.
[http://dx.doi.org/10.2337/diacare.24.6.1069] [PMID: 11375373]

[4]   Peyrot M, Rubin RR. Levels and risks of depression and anxiety symptomatology among diabetic adults. Diabetes Care 1997; 20(4): 585-90.
[http://dx.doi.org/10.2337/diacare.20.4.585] [PMID: 9096984]

[5]   Semenkovich K, Brown ME, Svrakic DM, Lustman PJ. Depression in type 2 diabetes mellitus: prevalence, impact, and treatment. Drugs 2015; 75(6): 577-87.
[http://dx.doi.org/10.1007/s40265-015-0347-4] [PMID: 25851098]

[6]   Ezzati M, Lopez AD, Rodgers A, Vander Hoorn S, Murray CJL. Selected major risk factors and global and regional burden of disease. Lancet 2002; 360(9343): 1347-60.
[http://dx.doi.org/10.1016/S0140-6736(02)11403-6] [PMID: 12423980]

[7]   Caballero B. The global epidemic of obesity: an overview. Epidemiol Rev 2007; 29(1): 1-5.
[http://dx.doi.org/10.1093/epirev/mxm012] [PMID: 17569676]

[8]   Abel ED, Peroni O, Kim JK, *et al.* Adipose-selective targeting of the GLUT4 gene impairs insulin action in muscle and liver 2001.
[http://dx.doi.org/10.1038/35055575]

[9]   Guilherme A, Virbasius JV, Puri V, Czech MP. Adipocyte dysfunctions linking obesity to insulin resistance and type 2 diabetes. Nat Rev Mol Cell Biol 2008; 9(5): 367-77.
[http://dx.doi.org/10.1038/nrm2391] [PMID: 18401346]

[10]   Rosen ED, Spiegelman BM. Adipocytes as regulators of energy balance and glucose homeostasis. Nature 2006; 444(7121): 847-53.
[http://dx.doi.org/10.1038/nature05483] [PMID: 17167472]

[11]   Hulver MW, Berggren JR, Cortright RN, *et al.* Skeletal muscle lipid metabolism with obesity. Am J Physiol Endocrinol Metab 2003; 284(4): E741-7.
[http://dx.doi.org/10.1152/ajpendo.00514.2002] [PMID: 12626325]

[12]   Kelley DE, Goodpaster B, Wing RR, Simoneau JA. Skeletal muscle fatty acid metabolism in association with insulin resistance, obesity, and weight loss. Am J Physiol 1999; 277(6): E1130-41.
[PMID: 10600804]

[13]   Li B, Nolte LA, Ju JS, *et al.* Skeletal muscle respiratory uncoupling prevents diet-induced obesity and insulin resistance in mice. Nat Med 2000; 6(10): 1115-20.
[http://dx.doi.org/10.1038/80450] [PMID: 11017142]

[14]   Jacka FN, Cherbuin N, Anstey KJ, Sachdev P, Butterworth P. Western diet is associated with a smaller hippocampus: a longitudinal investigation. BMC Med 2015; 13(1): 215.
[http://dx.doi.org/10.1186/s12916-015-0461-x] [PMID: 26349802]

[15]   Cherbuin N, Sargent-Cox K, Fraser M, Sachdev P, Anstey KJ. Being overweight is associated with hippocampal atrophy: the PATH Through Life Study. Int J Obes 2015; 39(10): 1509-14.
[http://dx.doi.org/10.1038/ijo.2015.106] [PMID: 26041696]

[16]   Jacka FN, Pasco JA, Mykletun A, *et al.* Association of Western and traditional diets with depression and anxiety in women. Am J Psychiatry 2010; 167(3): 305-11.
[http://dx.doi.org/10.1176/appi.ajp.2009.09060881] [PMID: 20048020]

[17]   Kan C, Silva N, Golden SH, *et al.* A systematic review and meta-analysis of the association between depression and insulin resistance. Diabetes Care 2013; 36(2): 480-9.
[http://dx.doi.org/10.2337/dc12-1442] [PMID: 23349152]

[18]   Skilton MR, Moulin P, Terra JL, Bonnet F. Associations between anxiety, depression, and the metabolic syndrome. Biol Psychiatry 2007; 62(11): 1251-7.
[http://dx.doi.org/10.1016/j.biopsych.2007.01.012] [PMID: 17553465]

[19]   Katon WJ, Rutter C, Simon G, *et al.* The association of comorbid depression with mortality in patients with type 2 diabetes. Diabetes Care 2005; 28(11): 2668-72.
[http://dx.doi.org/10.2337/diacare.28.11.2668] [PMID: 16249537]

[20]   Eaton WW, Armenian H, Gallo J, Pratt L, Ford DE. Depression and risk for onset of type II diabetes. A prospective population-based study. Diabetes Care 1996; 19(10): 1097-102.
[http://dx.doi.org/10.2337/diacare.19.10.1097] [PMID: 8886555]

[21]   Brown LC, Majumdar SR, Newman SC, Johnson JA. History of depression increases risk of type 2 diabetes in younger adults. Diabetes Care 2005; 28(5): 1063-7.
[http://dx.doi.org/10.2337/diacare.28.5.1063] [PMID: 15855568]

[22]   Shomaker LB, Tanofsky-Kraff M, Stern EA, *et al.* Longitudinal study of depressive symptoms and progression of insulin resistance in youth at risk for adult obesity. Diabetes Care 2011; 34(11): 2458-63.
[http://dx.doi.org/10.2337/dc11-1131] [PMID: 21911779]

[23]   Perry BI, Stochl J, Upthegrove R, *et al.* Longitudinal trends in childhood insulin levels and body mass index and associations with risks of psychosis and depression in young adults. JAMA Psychiatry 2021; 78(4): 416-25.
[http://dx.doi.org/10.1001/jamapsychiatry.2020.4180] [PMID: 33439216]

[24]   DeCarolis NA, Eisch AJ. Hippocampal neurogenesis as a target for the treatment of mental illness: A critical evaluation. Neuropharmacology 2010; 58(6): 884-93.
[http://dx.doi.org/10.1016/j.neuropharm.2009.12.013] [PMID: 20060007]

[25]   Altman J. Autoradiographic investigation of cell proliferation in the brains of rats and cats. Anat Rec 1963; 145(4): 573-91.
[http://dx.doi.org/10.1002/ar.1091450409] [PMID: 14012334]

[26]   Snyder JS, Soumier A, Brewer M, Pickel J, Cameron HA. Adult hippocampal neurogenesis buffers stress responses and depressive behaviour. Nature 2011; 476(7361): 458-61.
[http://dx.doi.org/10.1038/nature10287] [PMID: 21814201]

[27]   Brummelte S, Galea LAM. Chronic high corticosterone reduces neurogenesis in the dentate gyrus of adult male and female rats. Neuroscience 2010; 168(3): 680-90.
[http://dx.doi.org/10.1016/j.neuroscience.2010.04.023] [PMID: 20406669]

[28]   Malberg JE, Eisch AJ, Nestler EJ, Duman RS. Chronic antidepressant treatment increases neurogenesis in adult rat hippocampus. J Neurosci 2000; 20(24): 9104-10.
[http://dx.doi.org/10.1523/JNEUROSCI.20-24-09104.2000] [PMID: 11124987]

[29]   Wang JW, David DJ, Monckton JE, Battaglia F, Hen R. Chronic fluoxetine stimulates maturation and synaptic plasticity of adult-born hippocampal granule cells. J Neurosci 2008; 28(6): 1374-84.
[http://dx.doi.org/10.1523/JNEUROSCI.3632-07.2008] [PMID: 18256257]

[30]   Santarelli L, Saxe M, Gross C, *et al.* Requirement of hippocampal neurogenesis for the behavioral effects of antidepressants. Science 2003; 301(5634): 805-9.
[http://dx.doi.org/10.1126/science.1083328] [PMID: 12907793]

[31]   Nibuya M, Morinobu S, Duman RS. Regulation of BDNF and trkB mRNA in rat brain by chronic electroconvulsive seizure and antidepressant drug treatments. J Neurosci 1995; 15(11): 7539-47.
[http://dx.doi.org/10.1523/JNEUROSCI.15-11-07539.1995] [PMID: 7472505]

[32] Li Y, Luikart BW, Birnbaum S, *et al.* TrkB regulates hippocampal neurogenesis and governs sensitivity to antidepressive treatment. Neuron 2008; 59(3): 399-412.
[http://dx.doi.org/10.1016/j.neuron.2008.06.023] [PMID: 18701066]

[33] Almeida-Suhett CP, Graham A, Chen Y, Deuster P. Behavioral changes in male mice fed a high-fat diet are associated with IL-1β expression in specific brain regions. Physiol Behav 2017; 169: 130-40.
[http://dx.doi.org/10.1016/j.physbeh.2016.11.016] [PMID: 27876639]

[34] Sharma AN, Elased KM, Garrett TL, Lucot JB. Neurobehavioral deficits in *db/db* diabetic mice. Physiol Behav 2010; 101(3): 381-8.
[http://dx.doi.org/10.1016/j.physbeh.2010.07.002] [PMID: 20637218]

[35] Tomiga Y, Higaki Y, Anzai K, Takahashi H. Behavioral defects and downregulation of hippocampal BDNF and nNOS expression in db/db mice did not improved by chronic TGF-β2 treatment. Front Physiol 2022; 13: 969480. Epub ahead of print
[http://dx.doi.org/10.3389/fphys.2022.969480] [PMID: 36091357]

[36] Stranahan AM, Lee K, Martin B, *et al.* Voluntary exercise and caloric restriction enhance hippocampal dendritic spine density and BDNF levels in diabetic mice. Hippocampus 2009; 19(10): 951-61.
[http://dx.doi.org/10.1002/hipo.20577] [PMID: 19280661]

[37] Liu X, Yang LJ, Fan SJ, Jiang H, Pan F. Swimming exercise effects on the expression of HSP70 and iNOS in hippocampus and prefrontal cortex in combined stress. Neurosci Lett 2010; 476(2): 99-103.
[http://dx.doi.org/10.1016/j.neulet.2010.04.011] [PMID: 20398736]

[38] Molteni R, Barnard RJ, Ying Z, Roberts CK, Gómez-Pinilla F. A high-fat, refined sugar diet reduces hippocampal brain-derived neurotrophic factor, neuronal plasticity, and learning. Neuroscience 2002; 112(4): 803-14.
[http://dx.doi.org/10.1016/S0306-4522(02)00123-9] [PMID: 12088740]

[39] Park HR, Park M, Choi J, Park KY, Chung HY, Lee J. A high-fat diet impairs neurogenesis: Involvement of lipid peroxidation and brain-derived neurotrophic factor. Neurosci Lett 2010; 482(3): 235-9.
[http://dx.doi.org/10.1016/j.neulet.2010.07.046] [PMID: 20670674]

[40] Liu Y, Fu X, Lan N, *et al.* Luteolin protects against high fat diet-induced cognitive deficits in obesity mice. Behav Brain Res 2014; 267: 178-88.
[http://dx.doi.org/10.1016/j.bbr.2014.02.040] [PMID: 24667364]

[41] Hao S, Dey A, Yu X, Stranahan AM. Dietary obesity reversibly induces synaptic stripping by microglia and impairs hippocampal plasticity. Brain Behav Immun 2016; 51: 230-9.
[http://dx.doi.org/10.1016/j.bbi.2015.08.023] [PMID: 26336035]

[42] Robison LS, Albert NM, Camargo LA, *et al.* High-fat diet-induced obesity causes sex-specific deficits in adult hippocampal neurogenesis in mice. eNeuro 2020; 7(1): ENEURO.0391-19.2019. Epub ahead of print
[http://dx.doi.org/10.1523/ENEURO.0391-19.2019] [PMID: 31871124]

[43] Wosiski-Kuhn M, Erion JR, Gomez-Sanchez EP, Gomez-Sanchez CE, Stranahan AM. Glucocorticoid receptor activation impairs hippocampal plasticity by suppressing BDNF expression in obese mice. Psychoneuroendocrinology 2014; 42: 165-77.
[http://dx.doi.org/10.1016/j.psyneuen.2014.01.020] [PMID: 24636513]

[44] Fourrier C, Bosch-Bouju C, Boursereau R, *et al.* Brain tumor necrosis factor-α mediates anxiety-like behavior in a mouse model of severe obesity. Brain Behav Immun 2019; 77: 25-36.
[http://dx.doi.org/10.1016/j.bbi.2018.11.316] [PMID: 30508579]

[45] Bredt DS, Snyder SH. Transient nitric oxide synthase neurons in embryonic cerebral cortical plate, sensory ganglia, and olfactory epithelium. Neuron 1994; 13(2): 301-13.
[http://dx.doi.org/10.1016/0896-6273(94)90348-4] [PMID: 7520252]

[46] Abbott LC, Nahm SS. Neuronal nitric oxide synthase expression in cerebellar mutant mice.

Cerebellum 2004; 3(3): 141-51.
[http://dx.doi.org/10.1080/14734220410031927] [PMID: 15543804]

[47] Lüth HJ, Holzer M, Gertz HJ, Arendt T. Aberrant expression of nNOS in pyramidal neurons in Alzheimer's disease is highly co-localized with p21ras and p16INK4a. Brain Res 2000; 852(1): 45-55.
[http://dx.doi.org/10.1016/S0006-8993(99)02178-2] [PMID: 10661494]

[48] Zhou QG, Hu Y, Hua Y, *et al.* Neuronal nitric oxide synthase contributes to chronic stress-induced depression by suppressing hippocampal neurogenesis. J Neurochem 2007; 103(5): 1843-54.
[http://dx.doi.org/10.1111/j.1471-4159.2007.04914.x] [PMID: 17854383]

[49] Volke V, Wegener G, Bourin M, Vasar E. Antidepressant- and anxiolytic-like effects of selective neuronal NOS inhibitor 1-(2-trifluoromethylphenyl)-imidazole in mice. Behav Brain Res 2003; 140(1-2): 141-7.
[http://dx.doi.org/10.1016/S0166-4328(02)00312-1] [PMID: 12644287]

[50] Zhang J, Huang XY, Ye ML, *et al.* Neuronal nitric oxide synthase alteration accounts for the role of 5-HT1A receptor in modulating anxiety-related behaviors. J Neurosci 2010; 30(7): 2433-41.
[http://dx.doi.org/10.1523/JNEUROSCI.5880-09.2010] [PMID: 20164327]

[51] Tomiga Y, Yoshimura S, Ra SG, *et al.* Anxiety-like behaviors and hippocampal nNOS in response to diet-induced obesity combined with exercise. J Physiol Sci 2019; 69(5): 711-22.
[http://dx.doi.org/10.1007/s12576-019-00686-5] [PMID: 31124076]

[52] Tomiga Y, Yoshimura S, Ito A, *et al.* Exercise training rescues high fat diet-induced neuronal nitric oxide synthase expression in the hippocampus and cerebral cortex of mice. Nitric Oxide 2017; 66: 71-7.
[http://dx.doi.org/10.1016/j.niox.2017.03.002] [PMID: 28302517]

[53] Mikkelsen K, Stojanovska L, Polenakovic M, Bosevski M, Apostolopoulos V. Exercise and mental health. Maturitas 2017; 106: 48-56.
[http://dx.doi.org/10.1016/j.maturitas.2017.09.003] [PMID: 29150166]

[54] Northey JM, Cherbuin N, Pumpa KL, Smee DJ, Rattray B. Exercise interventions for cognitive function in adults older than 50: a systematic review with meta-analysis. Br J Sports Med 2018; 52(3): 154-60.
[http://dx.doi.org/10.1136/bjsports-2016-096587] [PMID: 28438770]

[55] Erickson KI, Voss MW, Prakash RS, *et al.* Exercise training increases size of hippocampus and improves memory. Proc Natl Acad Sci USA 2011; 108(7): 3017-22.
[http://dx.doi.org/10.1073/pnas.1015950108] [PMID: 21282661]

[56] Chang YK, Labban JD, Gapin JI, Etnier JL. The effects of acute exercise on cognitive performance: A meta-analysis. Brain Res 2012; 1453: 87-101.
[http://dx.doi.org/10.1016/j.brainres.2012.02.068] [PMID: 22480735]

[57] Tomporowski PD. Effects of acute bouts of exercise on cognition. Acta Psychol (Amst) 2003; 112(3): 297-324.
[http://dx.doi.org/10.1016/S0001-6918(02)00134-8] [PMID: 12595152]

[58] Bartholomew JB, Morrison D, Ciccolo JT. Effects of acute exercise on mood and well-being in patients with major depressive disorder. Med Sci Sports Exerc 2005; 37(12): 2032-7.
[http://dx.doi.org/10.1249/01.mss.0000178101.78322.dd] [PMID: 16331126]

[59] Ando S, Fujimoto T, Sudo M, *et al.* The neuromodulatory role of dopamine in improved reaction time by acute cardiovascular exercise. J Physiol 2024; 602(3): 461-84.
[http://dx.doi.org/10.1113/JP285173] [PMID: 38165254]

[60] Babyak M, Blumenthal JA, Herman S, *et al.* Exercise treatment for major depression: maintenance of therapeutic benefit at 10 months. Psychosom Med 2000; 62(5): 633-8.
[http://dx.doi.org/10.1097/00006842-200009000-00006] [PMID: 11020092]

[61] Neeper SA, Gómez-Pinilla F, Choi J, Cotman CW. Physical activity increases mRNA for brain-

derived neurotrophic factor and nerve growth factor in rat brain. Brain Res 1996; 726(1-2): 49-56.
[http://dx.doi.org/10.1016/0006-8993(96)00273-9] [PMID: 8836544]

[62]   Vaynman S, Ying Z, Gomez-Pinilla F. Hippocampal BDNF mediates the efficacy of exercise on synaptic plasticity and cognition. Eur J Neurosci 2004; 20(10): 2580-90.
[http://dx.doi.org/10.1111/j.1460-9568.2004.03720.x] [PMID: 15548201]

[63]   Adlard PA, Perreau VM, Cotman CW. The exercise-induced expression of BDNF within the hippocampus varies across life-span. Neurobiol Aging 2005; 26(4): 511-20.
[http://dx.doi.org/10.1016/j.neurobiolaging.2004.05.006] [PMID: 15653179]

[64]   Liu LL, Li JM, Su WJ, Wang B, Jiang CL. Sex differences in depressive-like behaviour may relate to imbalance of microglia activation in the hippocampus. Brain Behav Immun 2019; 81: 188-97.
[http://dx.doi.org/10.1016/j.bbi.2019.06.012] [PMID: 31181346]

[65]   Barha CK, Falck RS, Davis JC, Nagamatsu LS, Liu-Ambrose T. Sex differences in aerobic exercise efficacy to improve cognition: A systematic review and meta-analysis of studies in older rodents. Front Neuroendocrinol 2017; 46: 86-105.
[http://dx.doi.org/10.1016/j.yfrne.2017.06.001] [PMID: 28614695]

[66]   Barha CK, Liu-Ambrose T. Exercise and the aging brain: considerations for sex differences. Brain Plast 2018; 4(1): 53-63.
[http://dx.doi.org/10.3233/BPL-180067] [PMID: 30564546]

[67]   Tomiga Y, Sakai K, Ra SG, *et al.* Short-term running exercise alters DNA methylation patterns in neuronal nitric oxide synthase and brain-derived neurotrophic factor genes in the mouse hippocampus and reduces anxiety-like behaviors. FASEB J 2021; 35(8): e21767.
[http://dx.doi.org/10.1096/fj.202100630R] [PMID: 34325488]

[68]   Gomez-Pinilla F, Zhuang Y, Feng J, Ying Z, Fan G. Exercise impacts brain-derived neurotrophic factor plasticity by engaging mechanisms of epigenetic regulation. Eur J Neurosci 2011; 33(3): 383-90.
[http://dx.doi.org/10.1111/j.1460-9568.2010.07508.x] [PMID: 21198979]

[69]   Cai M, Wang H, Li J, *et al.* The signaling mechanisms of hippocampal endoplasmic reticulum stress affecting neuronal plasticity-related protein levels in high fat diet-induced obese rats and the regulation of aerobic exercise. Brain Behav Immun 2016; 57: 347-59.
[http://dx.doi.org/10.1016/j.bbi.2016.05.010] [PMID: 27189035]

[70]   Shima T, Matsui T, Jesmin S, *et al.* Moderate exercise ameliorates dysregulated hippocampal glycometabolism and memory function in a rat model of type 2 diabetes. Diabetologia 2017; 60(3): 597-606.
[http://dx.doi.org/10.1007/s00125-016-4164-4] [PMID: 27928614]

[71]   Wang P, Kong FZ, Hong XH, *et al.* Neuronal nitric oxide synthase regulates depression-like behaviors in shortening-induced obese mice. Nutrients 2022; 14(20): 4302.
[http://dx.doi.org/10.3390/nu14204302] [PMID: 36296987]

[72]   Pedersen BK, Saltin B. Exercise as medicine – evidence for prescribing exercise as therapy in 26 different chronic diseases. Scand J Med Sci Sports 2015; 25(S3) (Suppl. 3): 1-72.
[http://dx.doi.org/10.1111/sms.12581] [PMID: 26606383]

[73]   Pilegaard H, Saltin B, Neufer PD. Exercise induces transient transcriptional activation of the PGC-1α gene in human skeletal muscle. J Physiol 2003; 546(3): 851-8.
[http://dx.doi.org/10.1113/jphysiol.2002.034850] [PMID: 12563009]

[74]   Boström P, Wu J, Jedrychowski MP, *et al.* A PGC1-α-dependent myokine that drives brown-fat-like development of white fat and thermogenesis. Nature 2012; 481(7382): 463-8.
[http://dx.doi.org/10.1038/nature10777] [PMID: 22237023]

[75]   Tsuchiya Y, Ando D, Takamatsu K, Goto K. Resistance exercise induces a greater irisin response than endurance exercise. Metabolism 2015; 64(9): 1042-50.

[http://dx.doi.org/10.1016/j.metabol.2015.05.010] [PMID: 26081427]

[76]   Tsai CL, Pan CY, Tseng YT, Chen FC, Chang YC, Wang TC. Acute effects of high-intensity interval training and moderate-intensity continuous exercise on BDNF and irisin levels and neurocognitive performance in late middle-aged and older adults. Behav Brain Res 2021; 413: 113472.
        [http://dx.doi.org/10.1016/j.bbr.2021.113472] [PMID: 34274372]

[77]   Siteneski A, Olescowicz G, Pazini FL, *et al.* Antidepressant-like and pro-neurogenic effects of physical exercise: the putative role of FNDC5/irisin pathway. J Neural Transm (Vienna) 2020; 127(3): 355-70.
        [http://dx.doi.org/10.1007/s00702-020-02143-9] [PMID: 31974720]

[78]   Gruhn K, Siteneski A, Camargo A, *et al.* Physical exercise stimulates hippocampal mTORC1 and FNDC5/irisin signaling pathway in mice: Possible implication for its antidepressant effect. Behav Brain Res 2021; 400: 113040.
        [http://dx.doi.org/10.1016/j.bbr.2020.113040] [PMID: 33279634]

[79]   Wrann CD, White JP, Salogiannnis J, *et al.* Exercise induces hippocampal BDNF through a PGC-1α/FNDC5 pathway. Cell Metab 2013; 18(5): 649-59.
        [http://dx.doi.org/10.1016/j.cmet.2013.09.008] [PMID: 24120943]

[80]   Islam MR, Valaris S, Young MF, *et al.* Exercise hormone irisin is a critical regulator of cognitive function. Nat Metab 2021; 3(8): 1058-70.
        [http://dx.doi.org/10.1038/s42255-021-00438-z] [PMID: 34417591]

[81]   Moon HY, Becke A, Berron D, *et al.* Running-induced systemic cathepsin b secretion is associated with memory function. Cell Metab 2016; 24(2): 332-40.
        [http://dx.doi.org/10.1016/j.cmet.2016.05.025] [PMID: 27345423]

[82]   El Hayek L, Khalifeh M, Zibara V, *et al.* Lactate mediates the effects of exercise on learning and memory through SIRT1-dependent activation of hippocampal brain-derived neurotrophic factor (BDNF). J Neurosci 2019; 39(13): 1661-18.
        [http://dx.doi.org/10.1523/JNEUROSCI.1661-18.2019] [PMID: 30692222]

[83]   Tran TT, Yamamoto Y, Gesta S, Kahn CR. Beneficial effects of subcutaneous fat transplantation on metabolism. Cell Metab 2008; 7(5): 410-20.
        [http://dx.doi.org/10.1016/j.cmet.2008.04.004] [PMID: 18460332]

[84]   Stanford KI, Middelbeek RJW, Townsend KL, *et al.* A novel role for subcutaneous adipose tissue in exercise-induced improvements in glucose homeostasis. Diabetes 2015; 64(6): 2002-14.
        [http://dx.doi.org/10.2337/db14-0704] [PMID: 25605808]

[85]   Takahashi H, Alves CRR, Stanford KI, *et al.* TGF-β2 is an exercise-induced adipokine that regulates glucose and fatty acid metabolism. Nat Metab 2019; 1(2): 291-303.
        [http://dx.doi.org/10.1038/s42255-018-0030-7] [PMID: 31032475]

CHAPTER 5

Muscle Atrophy and Weakness in Metabolic Disease

Hiroaki Eshima[1,*]

[1] *Department of International Tourism, Sports Tourism Course, Nagasaki International University, Nagasaki, Japan*

Abstract: Obesity and diabetes are associated with changes in skeletal muscle quantity and quality, such as increased ectopic fat, muscle atrophy, and decreased muscle strength. Skeletal muscle tissue is often affected by metabolic insult because it remodels cellular size, composition, and function in response to a variety of nutritional changes. Declining muscle quantity and quality are directly linked to falls and bedriddenness; understanding the intracellular mechanisms may provide clues for therapeutic strategies. How metabolic diseases *via* cellular mechanisms affect muscle quality and muscle quantity are presented in this chapter.

Keywords: Contraction, Calcium, Diabetes, Fiber type, Motor neuron, Myofibrillar, Obesity, Skeletal muscle, Satellite cell.

INTRODUCTION

Skeletal muscle is one of the largest organs in humans and accounts for ~40% of body mass in healthy-weight individuals, which is important for maintaining metabolic health [1]. Carbohydrates and fats are the primary nutrients that provide the necessary energy required during exercise. However, the metabolic insults in the regulation of glucose and lipids cause skeletal muscle abnormalities. As fat increases in the body due to lipid accumulation, the risk of type 2 diabetes mellitus (T2DM) increases, which is associated with insulin resistance in skeletal muscle [2]. Previous studies have focused on the cellular and molecular mechanisms of obesity- and diabetes-induced insulin resistance in skeletal muscle. On the other hand, recent studies have focused on the effect metabolic insult has on the loss of muscle size, strength, and physical function.

Skeletal muscle tissues are heterogeneous in their composition and mainly divided into slow-twitch and fast-twitch myofibers. The differences between slow- and

---

[*] **Corresponding author Hiroaki Eshima:** Department of International Tourism, Sports Tourism Course, Nagasaki International University, Nagasaki, Japan; E-mail: heshima@niu.ac.jp

Hiroaki Eshima, Ikuru Miura, Yutaka Matsunaga & Yuki Tomiga (Eds.)

fast-twitch fibers are the contractile proteins and types of energy metabolism, such as ATP production from mitochondria [3]. Furthermore, skeletal muscle adapts to numerous stimuli such as exercise, nutrition, disease, and aging, and these responses are manifested through changes in muscle size, fiber-type distribution, and metabolism. In contrast, muscle atrophy and weakness decrease the quality of life and increase the risk of injuries, falls, and the development of diseases. Indeed, diabetes and obesity cause loss of muscle mass and decrease muscle strength [4, 5]. Pharmacologic therapy for muscle loss induced by metabolic disease does not exist, and current diet/exercise therapeutic approaches are often ineffective and/or unfeasible.

This chapter will address skeletal muscle metabolism in metabolic disease through a brief comprehensive summary and describe the potential mechanisms of dysfunction of contractile force (weakness) and muscle atrophy induced by metabolic disease in skeletal muscle.

MUSCLE ATROPHY IN METABOLIC DISEASE

Lipids often ectopically accumulate in non-adipose tissues, including skeletal muscle [6]. Muscle lipids have been extensively studied in the context of metabolism, such as insulin sensitivity [7 - 9]. However, muscle lipid overload appears to affect not only metabolism but also muscle quantity, such as muscle maintenance and regeneration. There is evidence that diabetic myopathy is unfavorable for muscle growth and regeneration [10 - 12]. The loss of muscle mass in metabolic disorders is partly accounted for by an altered balance between synthesis and degradation in protein [13, 14]. Previous studies have reported that obesity causes the loss of muscle mass due to a decrease in muscle protein synthase and activation of protein degradation [15 - 17]. On the other hand, a high-fat diet (HFD) does not change the muscle protein synthase [18]. The lipid overload increases protein synthesis in skeletal muscle in rodent models [19]. These findings suggest that the mechanism underlying the muscle atrophy in metabolic disorders has not been fully elucidated.

Mechanisms that may contribute to lower muscle mass of metabolic disease can include decreases in the satellite cell. A previous study has reported that the differentiation of myoblasts is impaired in patients with diabetes, suggesting that one of the underlying causes of muscle loss [20]. Diabetic myoblasts had a reduced ability to differentiate into skeletal muscles, whereas administration of myogenic oligodeoxynucleotide improved skeletal muscle differentiation exacerbated by diabetes [20]. In obese rodent models, obese Zucker rats reduce the number of satellite cells, which may be a factor that contributes to the reduced muscle mass [12]. Interestingly, satellite cell proliferation can be restored with compensatory loading with surgery. Similar results were obtained in mice models of T2DM, and impaired muscle regeneration in T2DM mice was associated with reduced accumulation of macrophage and angiogenesis [21]. This cytokine was increased in muscle in patients with T2DM, suggesting a possible mechanism by which muscle function is compromised in diabetes [22]. These findings suggest that metabolic disease severity will mainly influence the functions of satellite cells.

Insulin resistance is associated with increased lipolysis and the release of free fatty acids from adipose tissue, which may lead to the inhibition of muscle regeneration through the growth hormone/insulin growth factor-1 [5, 23]. Furthermore, oxidative stress, mitochondrial dysfunction, inflammation, and protein degradation pathways have been implicated in muscle atrophy and weakness. Indeed, these factors are increased in skeletal muscle of metabolic diseases [24]. For example, metformin is a commonly prescribed medication for T2DM patients due to decreased hepatic glucose production and intestinal absorption of glucose. A previous study showed that metformin ameliorates muscle atrophy due to decreased muscle atrophy-related genes in HFD-induced obese rats [25]. However, a long-term administration of metformin causes accelerates muscle atrophy through the activation of phosphorylated AMPK in *db/db* mice [26]. Metformin should be prescribed to patients with T2DM because of its great efficacy in reducing hyperglycemia and other diabetes-related complications, but there is no effective treatment for muscle wasting that has been established. Metformin might induce muscle atrophy that is regulated in an AMPK-dependent manner [27 - 30]. AMPK is not only associated with the glucose transporter system but also inhibits anabolic processes such as protein synthesis and increases protein degradation and autophagy [31]. Thus, it is skeptical whether antidiabetic drugs are necessarily effective against muscle atrophy.

MUSCLE CONTRACTILE ADAPTATION IN METABOLIC DISEASE

Rodent studies demonstrate that obesity induced by HFD impairs contractile function with electrical stimulation, enhanced fatigability, and increased muscle fragility [32 - 34]. A previous study demonstrated that middle-aged mice fed HFD exhibited decreased grip strength [35]. Consistent with this, another study also shows that the contractile force was lower in aged mice fed HFD [36]. These findings suggest that the synergistic effects of obesity and aging may exacerbate muscle contractile dysfunction. Consistent with these findings, Eshima *et al.* recently demonstrated that chronic HFD feeding significantly reduced contractile force in fast-twitch dominant muscles but not slow-twitch dominant muscle in aged skeletal muscle [33] (Fig. **1**).

Diabetes often causes muscle atrophy and weakness, and it is called "diabetic myopathy," like sarcopenia [37, 38]. Metabolic diseases, including obesity and T2DM, may undergo alteration in muscle fiber types. Fast-twitch glycolytic (myosin-heavy chain (MyHC) type II fibers have contributed to force production rather than slow-twitch oxidative (MyHC type I fibers). Diabetes and obesity increase the relative percentage of MyHC type I and decrease that of MyHC type II fibers [34, 39 - 43]. Muscle contractile force largely depends on fiber type and metabolic profile of mammalian skeletal muscle [44, 45]. Hence, muscle contractile dysfunction in metabolic disease may contribute to different fiber types (Fig. **2**).

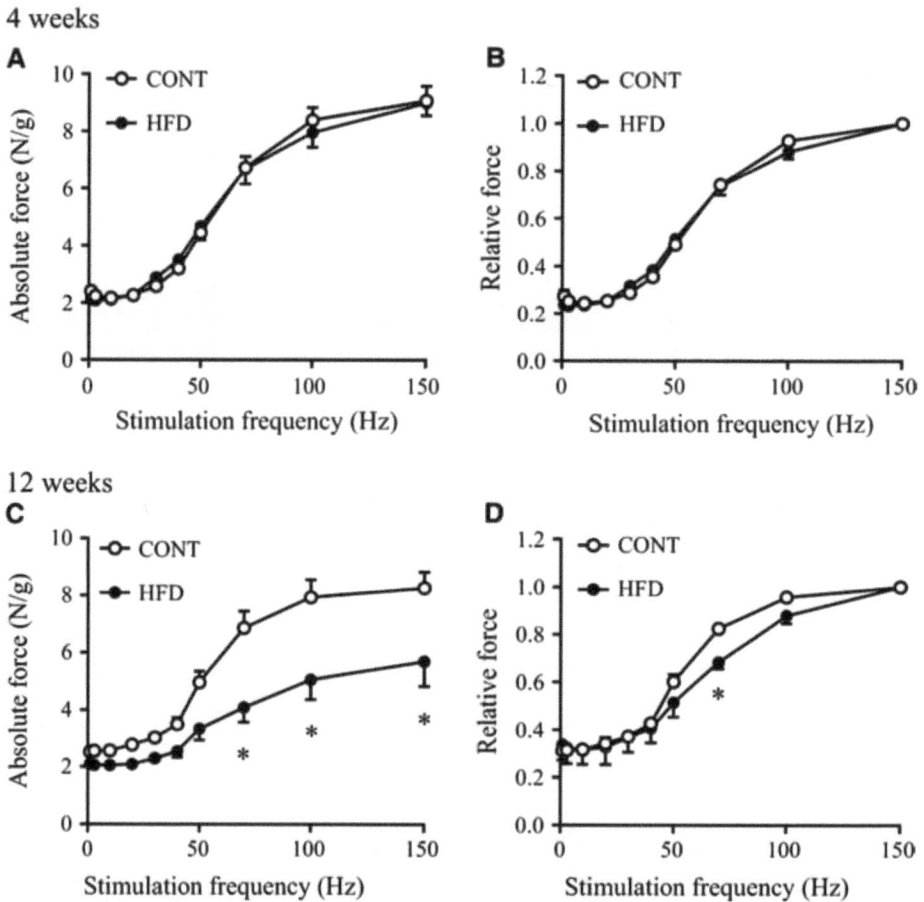

Fig. (1). Force production in fast-twitch dominant muscles was lower in mice fed a high-fat diet (HFD). Isometric tension at several frequencies was determined in fast-twitch dominant muscles from control (CONT) and HFD-fed mice. Absolute force per muscle mass (A: 4 weeks; C: 12 weeks) and relative force calculated by each value normalized to the maximum force. From [34].

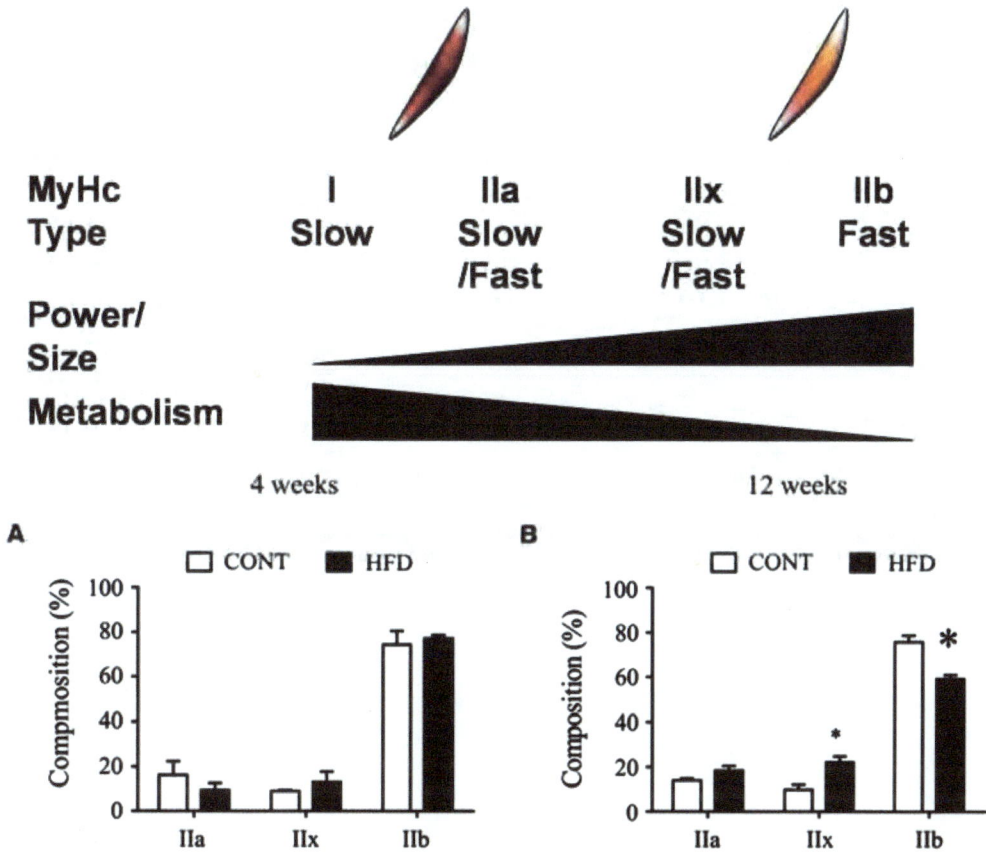

Fig. (2). Morphometric changes of muscles after a high-fat diet (HFD). Schematic diagram of the muscle fiber type. Myosin heavy chains (MyHc) are classified into four types: I, IIa, IIx, and IIb. In EDL muscles from the 12-week HFD group, but not the 4-week HFD group, there was an increased percentage of MHC type IIa/x fibers, mainly at the expense of decreased type IIb fibers. From [34].

Muscle contraction is regulated by intracellular signaling. An excitable membrane has a stable potential when there is no net ion current flowing across the membrane. However, action potentials originate after a muscle cell is depolarized to threshold propagate along the skeletal muscle membrane [46]. The muscle fibers repolarize and induce action potentials when the external calcium concentration is raised, resulting in the effects of changes in extracellular calcium (Ca^{2+}) upon properties [47]. Ca^{2+} binds to troponin and permits actin-myosin interaction. The heads of myosin are detached as long as tropomyosin impedes the interaction of actin and myosin but will undergo cycles of binding and exerting force when the binding of Ca^{2+} to troponin results in the movement of tropomyosin to a position [48]. Thus, Ca^{2+} is important cellular signaling for muscle contraction (Fig. **3**). Ca^{2+} is a highly versatile intracellular signal in living tissue and regulates cellular processes that function over a wide range [49] (Fig. **4**). In skeletal muscle, the deficit of contractile function is impairments of calcium cycling known as excitation-contraction coupling. In fact, dysregulation of Ca^{2+} release from the sarcoplasmic reticulum (SR) has been reported in obese and diabetic skeletal muscles [33, 50]. Consistent with this finding, previous studies demonstrate impaired Ca^{2+} release during muscle contraction in obese [51] and diabetic mice [52]. These results suggest that dysfunctional Ca^{2+} flux may contribute to contractile dysfunction in metabolic disease. However, another study showed no differences in calcium cycling between healthy muscle and obese muscle [53].

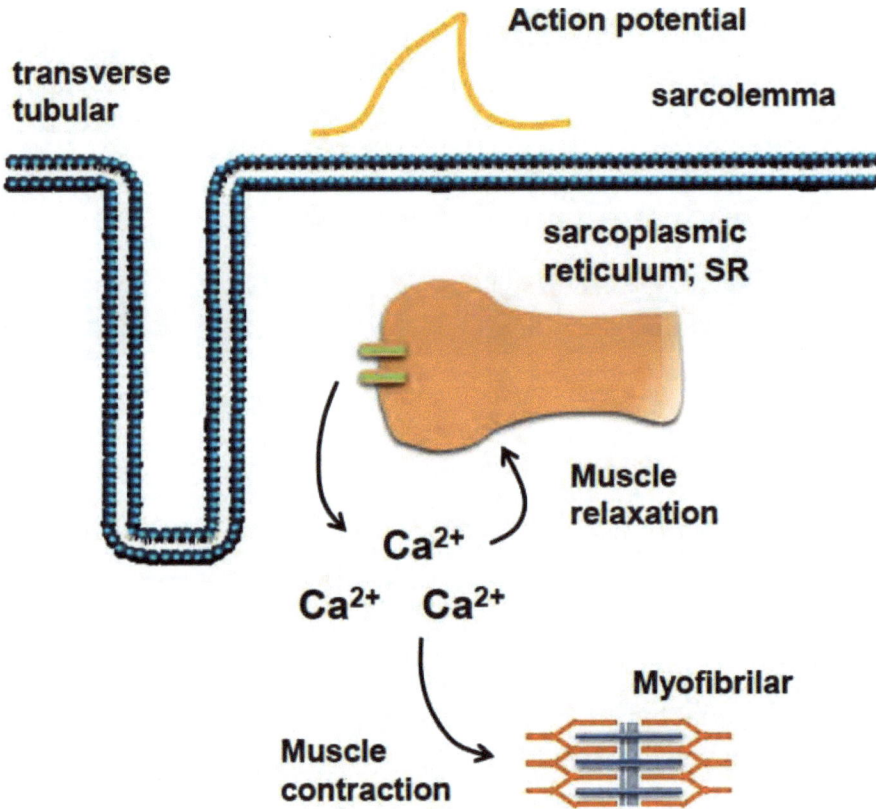

Fig. (3). Cellular and molecular mechanisms of muscle contraction.

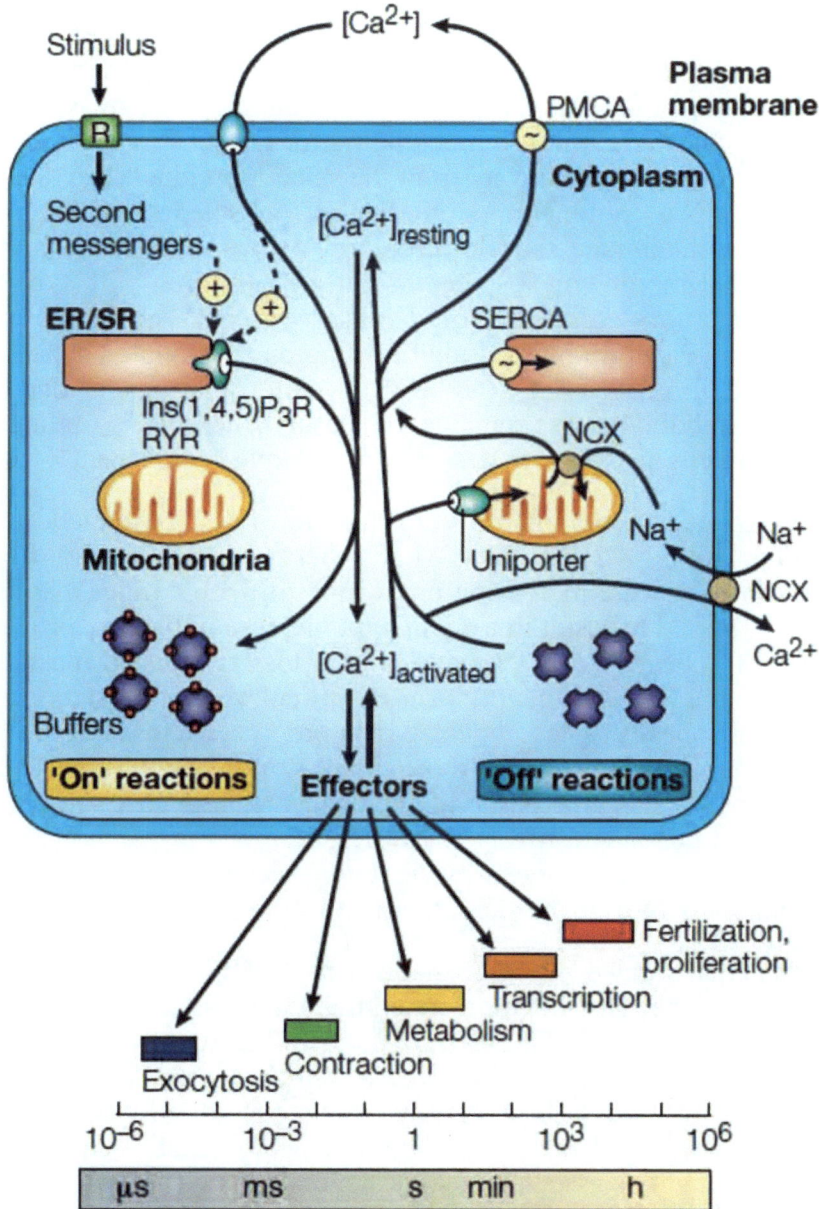

Fig. (4). The dynamics and homeostasis of calcium. During the 'on' reactions, stimuli induce both the entry of external Ca^{2+} and the formation of second messengers that release internal Ca^{2+} that is stored in the endoplasmic/sarcoplasmic reticulum (ER/SR). Most of this Ca^{2+} is bound to buffers, but a small proportion binds to the effectors that activate various cellular processes that operate over a wide temporal spectrum. During the 'off' reactions, Ca^{2+} leaves the effectors and buffers and is removed from the cell by various exchangers and pumps. From [49].

During stimulation, stimuli induce both the entry of external Ca^{2+} and the formation of second messengers that release an accelerated loss of motor neurons, which may underlie the accelerated loss of muscle strength with metabolic diseases. This association establishes such a link and requires an assessment of the number of muscle fibers, motor units, and motor neurons in the spinal cord that innervate the muscles in the lower leg in the same individual. Diabetes causes an early loss of alpha motoneurons in skeletal muscles, and loss of gamma motoneurons might induce muscle atrophy [54]. In humans, a previous study demonstrates that motor unit loss begins early in children with type 1 diabetes [55]. Indeed, neuromuscular junction damage was observed in obese mice, and the impacts of a long-term high-fat diet feeding obesity-related synaptic changes were identified [56]. Whether the loss of motor neurons is due to muscle weakness in metabolic disease remains to be established; these findings may thus inform interventions and policies designed to improve health span.

The chronic overconsumption of Western-style diets has long been a leading cause of obesity and T2DM [57, 58]. Furthermore, this is significant as the obesity epidemic and the increasing proportion of people older than 65 years in the world is expected to result in a significant increase in the proportion of people with sarcopenic obesity [59]. The age-related loss of muscle mass contributes significantly to the impaired quality of life, particularly during sarcopenic obesity [60]. Sarcopenic obesity is accompanied by a progressive loss of muscle function that causes mobility limitations more than sarcopenia alone. The mobility limitations impair accustomed mobility and cause a premature transition from an independent to a dependent lifestyle. Hence, there is a pressing need to develop interventions and/or encourage lifestyle changes that reverse, or even prevent, muscle weakness in old age, particularly in obesity.

In the fundamental studies, old mice that consumed HFD exhibited decreased grip strength [35]. Another study demonstrated that the contractile force was lower in old mice that had consumed HFD [61]. These studies suggest that the synergistic effects of obesity and aging may exacerbate contractile dysfunction. Eshima *et al.* demonstrated that chronic HFD significantly reduced contractile force in aged mice [33]. Consistent with this finding, contractile dysfunction in obese and aging skeletal muscle might be associated with calcium cycling (Fig. **5**).

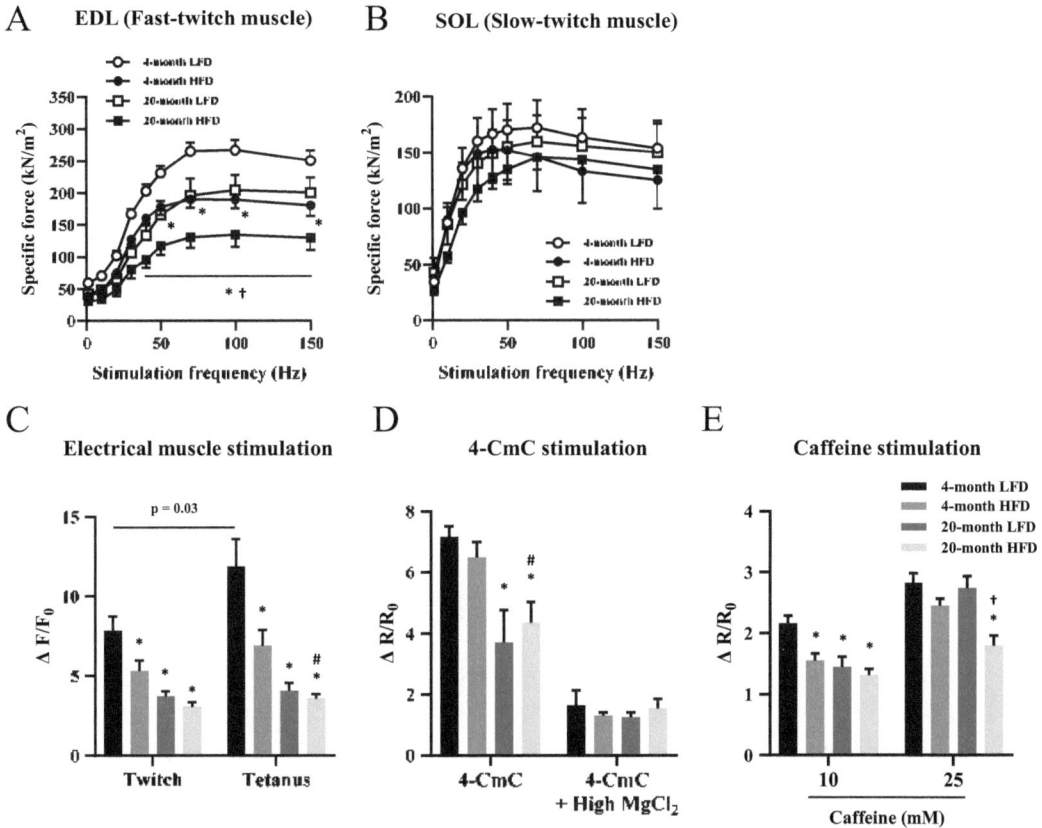

Fig. (5). Chronic high-fat diet (20 months) accelerates muscle weakness in fast-twitch dominant muscles (**A**) but not slow-twitch dominant muscles (**B**), in aged mice. Average peak Ca^{2+} responses (fluo-4 fluorescence) during twitch and tetanus stimulation (**C**). Average peak Ca^{2+} responses (fura-2 fluorescence) during 4-chloro-m-cresol (4-CmC) with or without 30 mM MgCl stimulation (**D**). Average peak Ca^{2+} responses (fura-2 fluorescence) in the presence of low and high concentrations of caffeine (D). LFD: low-fat diet, HFD: high-fat diet. *p < 0.05 *vs*. 4-month LFD. †p < 0.05 *vs*. 4-month HFD and 20-month LFD. Values shown are the means ± SE. From [33].

To inform such interventions and/or lifestyle changes, a fundamental understanding of the cause of muscle weakness is essential. Taken together, we summarize the potential mechanism for loss of muscle mass and impaired contractile function in skeletal muscles of metabolic diseases such as obese and T2DM animals and patients see Fig. (**6**).

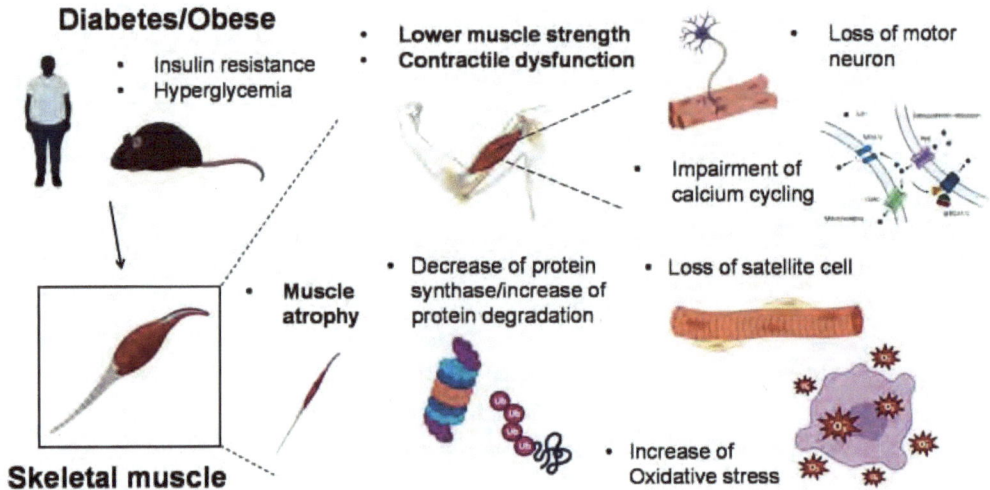

Fig. (6). Schematic diagram of the potential cellular mechanisms for loss of muscle mass and impaired contractile function in metabolic diseases.

CONCLUDING REMARKS

This chapter considered the impact of metabolic disorders, such as obesity and type 2 diabetes, on morphology and function in skeletal muscle. The potential mechanism of loss of muscle mass and contractile dysfunction in metabolic disorders has not been fully clarified. If future studies allow us to determine potential cellular mechanisms, they may provide clues for therapeutic strategies to promote skeletal muscle health and improve the overall quality of life.

REFERENCES

[1]   Baskin KK, Winders BR, Olson EN. Muscle as a "mediator" of systemic metabolism. Cell Metab 2015; 21(2): 237-48.
        [http://dx.doi.org/10.1016/j.cmet.2014.12.021] [PMID: 25651178]

[2]   Newman AB, Kupelian V, Visser M, *et al*. Strength, but not muscle mass, is associated with mortality in the health, aging and body composition study cohort. J Gerontol A Biol Sci Med Sci 2006; 61(1): 72-7.
        [http://dx.doi.org/10.1093/gerona/61.1.72] [PMID: 16456196]

[3]   Schiaffino S, Reggiani C. Fiber types in mammalian skeletal muscles. Physiol Rev 2011; 91(4): 1447-531.
        [http://dx.doi.org/10.1152/physrev.00031.2010] [PMID: 22013216]

[4]   Nomura T, Kawae T, Kataoka H, Ikeda Y. Assessment of lower extremity muscle mass, muscle strength, and exercise therapy in elderly patients with diabetes mellitus. Environ Health Prev Med 2018; 23(1): 20.
        [http://dx.doi.org/10.1186/s12199-018-0710-7] [PMID: 29776338]

[5]   Kalyani RR, Corriere M, Ferrucci L. Age-related and disease-related muscle loss: the effect of diabetes, obesity, and other diseases. Lancet Diabetes Endocrinol 2014; 2(10): 819-29.
        [http://dx.doi.org/10.1016/S2213-8587(14)70034-8] [PMID: 24731660]

[6]   Unger RH, Clark GO, Scherer PE, Orci L. Lipid homeostasis, lipotoxicity and the metabolic syndrome. Biochim Biophys Acta Mol Cell Biol Lipids 2010; 1801(3): 209-14.
[http://dx.doi.org/10.1016/j.bbalip.2009.10.006] [PMID: 19948243]

[7]   Funai K, Lodhi IJ, Spears LD, *et al.* Skeletal muscle phospholipid metabolism regulates insulin sensitivity and contractile function. Diabetes 2016; 65(2): 358-70.
[http://dx.doi.org/10.2337/db15-0659] [PMID: 26512026]

[8]   Lodhi IJ, Yin L, Jensen-Urstad APL, *et al.* Inhibiting adipose tissue lipogenesis reprograms thermogenesis and PPARγ activation to decrease diet-induced obesity. Cell Metab 2012; 16(2): 189-201.
[http://dx.doi.org/10.1016/j.cmet.2012.06.013] [PMID: 22863804]

[9]   Funai K, Song H, Yin L, *et al.* Muscle lipogenesis balances insulin sensitivity and strength through calcium signaling. J Clin Invest 2013; 123(3): 1229-40.
[http://dx.doi.org/10.1172/JCI65726] [PMID: 23376793]

[10]   Krause MP, Riddell MC, Gordon CS, Imam SA, Cafarelli E, Hawke TJ. Diabetic myopathy differs between Ins2Akita+/- and streptozotocin-induced Type 1 diabetic models. J Appl Physiol 1985; 2009(106): 1650-9.

[11]   Krause MP, Moradi J, Nissar AA, Riddell MC, Hawke TJ. Inhibition of plasminogen activator inhibitor-1 restores skeletal muscle regeneration in untreated type 1 diabetic mice. Diabetes 2011; 60(7): 1964-72.
[http://dx.doi.org/10.2337/db11-0007] [PMID: 21593201]

[12]   Peterson JM, Bryner RW, Alway SE. Satellite cell proliferation is reduced in muscles of obese Zucker rats but restored with loading. Am J Physiol Cell Physiol 2008; 295(2): C521-8.
[http://dx.doi.org/10.1152/ajpcell.00073.2008] [PMID: 18508911]

[13]   Argilés JM, Busquets S, Alvarez B, López-Soriano FJ. Mechanism for the increased skeletal muscle protein degradation in the obese zucker rat. J Nutr Biochem 1999; 10(4): 244-8.
[http://dx.doi.org/10.1016/S0955-2863(98)00098-9] [PMID: 15539297]

[14]   Durschlag RP, Layman DK. Skeletal muscle growth in lean and obese Zucker rats. Growth 1983; 47(3): 282-91.
[PMID: 6196256]

[15]   Lipina C, Hundal HS. Lipid modulation of skeletal muscle mass and function. J Cachexia Sarcopenia Muscle 2017; 8(2): 190-201.
[http://dx.doi.org/10.1002/jcsm.12144] [PMID: 27897400]

[16]   Tsintzas K, Jones R, Pabla P, *et al.* Effect of acute and short-term dietary fat ingestion on postprandial skeletal muscle protein synthesis rates in middle-aged, overweight, and obese men. Am J Physiol Endocrinol Metab 2020; 318(3): E417-29.
[http://dx.doi.org/10.1152/ajpendo.00344.2019] [PMID: 31910028]

[17]   Sishi B, Loos B, Ellis B, Smith W, du Toit EF, Engelbrecht AM. Diet-induced obesity alters signalling pathways and induces atrophy and apoptosis in skeletal muscle in a prediabetic rat model. Exp Physiol 2011; 96(2): 179-93.
[http://dx.doi.org/10.1113/expphysiol.2010.054189] [PMID: 20952489]

[18]   Estornell E, Cabo J, Barber T. Protein synthesis is stimulated in nutritionally obese rats. J Nutr 1995; 125(5): 1309-15.
[PMID: 7537806]

[19]   Estornell E, Barber T, Cabo J. Protein synthesis *in vivo* in rats fed on lipid-rich liquid diets. Br J Nutr 1994; 72(4): 509-17.
[http://dx.doi.org/10.1079/BJN19940055] [PMID: 7527251]

[20]   Nakamura S, Yonekura S, Shimosato T, Takaya T. Myogenetic oligodeoxynucleotide (myoDN) recovers the differentiation of skeletal muscle myoblasts deteriorated by diabetes mellitus. Front

Physiol 2021; 12: 679152.
[http://dx.doi.org/10.3389/fphys.2021.679152] [PMID: 34108889]

[21] Nguyen MH, Cheng M, Koh TJ. Impaired muscle regeneration in ob/ob and db/db mice. ScientificWorldJournal 2011; 11: 1525-35.
[http://dx.doi.org/10.1100/tsw.2011.137] [PMID: 21805021]

[22] Broholm C, Brandt C, Schultz NS, Nielsen AR, Pedersen BK, Scheele C. Deficient leukemia inhibitory factor signaling in muscle precursor cells from patients with type 2 diabetes. Am J Physiol Endocrinol Metab 2012; 303(2): E283-92.
[http://dx.doi.org/10.1152/ajpendo.00586.2011] [PMID: 22649064]

[23] Postic C, Girard J. Contribution of *de novo* fatty acid synthesis to hepatic steatosis and insulin resistance: lessons from genetically engineered mice. J Clin Invest 2008; 118(3): 829-38.
[http://dx.doi.org/10.1172/JCI34275] [PMID: 18317565]

[24] Shen Y, Li M, Wang K, *et al.* Diabetic muscular atrophy: molecular mechanisms and promising therapies. Front Endocrinol (Lausanne) 2022; 13: 917113.
[http://dx.doi.org/10.3389/fendo.2022.917113] [PMID: 35846289]

[25] Hasan MM, Shalaby SM, El-Gendy J, Abdelghany EMA. Beneficial effects of metformin on muscle atrophy induced by obesity in rats. J Cell Biochem 2019; 120(4): 5677-86.
[http://dx.doi.org/10.1002/jcb.27852] [PMID: 30320911]

[26] Kang MJ, Moon JW, Lee JO, *et al.* Metformin induces muscle atrophy by transcriptional regulation of myostatin *via* HDAC6 and FoxO3a. J Cachexia Sarcopenia Muscle 2022; 13(1): 605-20.
[http://dx.doi.org/10.1002/jcsm.12833] [PMID: 34725961]

[27] Das AK, Yang QY, Fu X, *et al.* AMP-activated protein kinase stimulates myostatin expression in C2C12 cells. Biochem Biophys Res Commun 2012; 427(1): 36-40.
[http://dx.doi.org/10.1016/j.bbrc.2012.08.138] [PMID: 22995402]

[28] De Lima EA, de Sousa LGO, de S Teixeira AA, Marshall AG, Zanchi NE, Neto JCR. Aerobic exercise, but not metformin, prevents reduction of muscular performance by AMPk activation in mice on doxorubicin chemotherapy. J Cell Physiol 2018; 233(12): 9652-62.
[http://dx.doi.org/10.1002/jcp.26880] [PMID: 29953589]

[29] De Fatima Silva F, Ortiz-Silva M, Galia WBS, *et al.* Effects of metformin on insulin resistance and metabolic disorders in tumor-bearing rats with advanced cachexia. Can J Physiol Pharmacol 2018; 96(5): 498-505.
[http://dx.doi.org/10.1139/cjpp-2017-0171] [PMID: 29304290]

[30] Krawiec BJ, Nystrom GJ, Frost RA, Jefferson LS, Lang CH. AMP-activated protein kinase agonists increase mRNA content of the muscle-specific ubiquitin ligases MAFbx and MuRF1 in C_2C_{12} cells. Am J Physiol Endocrinol Metab 2007; 292(6): E1555-67.
[http://dx.doi.org/10.1152/ajpendo.00622.2006] [PMID: 17264220]

[31] Thomson DM. The role of AMPK in the regulation of skeletal muscle size, hypertrophy, and regeneration. Int J Mol Sci 2018; 19(10): 3125.
[http://dx.doi.org/10.3390/ijms19103125] [PMID: 30314396]

[32] Yamamoto H, Eshima H, Kakehi S, Kawamori R, Watada H, Tamura Y. Impaired fatigue resistance, sarcoplasmic reticulum function, and mitochondrial activity in soleus muscle of db/db mice. Physiol Rep 2022; 10(18): e15478.
[http://dx.doi.org/10.14814/phy2.15478] [PMID: 36117307]

[33] Eshima H, Tamura Y, Kakehi S, *et al.* A chronic high-fat diet exacerbates contractile dysfunction with impaired intracellular Ca^{2+} release capacity in the skeletal muscle of aged mice. J Appl Physiol 2020; 128(5): 1153-62.
[http://dx.doi.org/10.1152/japplphysiol.00530.2019] [PMID: 32213111]

[34] Eshima H, Tamura Y, Kakehi S, *et al.* Long-term, but not short-term high-fat diet induces fiber

composition changes and impaired contractile force in mouse fast-twitch skeletal muscle. Physiol Rep 2017; 5(7): e13250.
[http://dx.doi.org/10.14814/phy2.13250] [PMID: 28408640]

[35] Lee SR, Khamoui AV, Jo E, *et al.* Effects of chronic high-fat feeding on skeletal muscle mass and function in middle-aged mice. Aging Clin Exp Res 2015; 27(4): 403-11.
[http://dx.doi.org/10.1007/s40520-015-0316-5] [PMID: 25647784]

[36] Abrigo J, Rivera JC, Aravena J, *et al.* High fat diet-induced skeletal muscle wasting is decreased by mesenchymal stem cells administration: implications on oxidative stress, ubiquitin proteasome pathway activation, and myonuclear apoptosis. Oxid Med Cell Longev 2016; 2016(1): 9047821.
[http://dx.doi.org/10.1155/2016/9047821] [PMID: 27579157]

[37] Eshima H, Poole DC, Kano Y. *In vivo* calcium regulation in diabetic skeletal muscle. Cell Calcium 2014; 56(5): 381-9.
[http://dx.doi.org/10.1016/j.ceca.2014.08.008] [PMID: 25224503]

[38] Perry BD, Caldow MK, Brennan-Speranza TC, *et al.* Muscle atrophy in patients with Type 2 Diabetes Mellitus: roles of inflammatory pathways, physical activity and exercise. Exerc Immunol Rev 2016; 22: 94-109.
[PMID: 26859514]

[39] Klueber KM, Feczko JD. Ultrastructural, histochemical, and morphometric analysis of skeletal muscle in a murine model of type I diabetes. Anat Rec 1994; 239(1): 18-34.
[http://dx.doi.org/10.1002/ar.1092390104] [PMID: 8037375]

[40] Jerković R, Bosnar A, Jurisić-Erzen D, *et al.* The effects of long-term experimental diabetes mellitus type I on skeletal muscle regeneration capacity. Coll Antropol 2009; 33(4): 1115-9.
[PMID: 20102056]

[41] Klueber KM, Feczko JD, Schmidt G, Watkins JB III. Skeletal muscle in the diabetic mouse: Histochemical and morphometric analysis. Anat Rec 1989; 225(1): 41-5.
[http://dx.doi.org/10.1002/ar.1092250107] [PMID: 2774212]

[42] Eshima H, Poole DC, Kano Y. *In vivo* Ca^{2+} buffering capacity and microvascular oxygen pressures following muscle contractions in diabetic rat skeletal muscles: fiber-type specific effects. Am J Physiol Regul Integr Comp Physiol 2015; 309(2): R128-37.
[http://dx.doi.org/10.1152/ajpregu.00044.2015] [PMID: 25947169]

[43] Tagawa T, Eshima H, Kakehi S, Kawamori R, Watada H, Tamura Y. A chronic high-fat diet does not exacerbate muscle atrophy in fast-twitch skeletal muscle of aged mice. Exp Physiol 2023; 108(7): 940-5.
[http://dx.doi.org/10.1113/EP091106] [PMID: 37074636]

[44] Bárány M. ATPase activity of myosin correlated with speed of muscle shortening. J Gen Physiol 1967; 50(6) (Suppl.): 197-218.
[http://dx.doi.org/10.1085/jgp.50.6.197] [PMID: 4227924]

[45] Baylor SM, Hollingworth S. Sarcoplasmic reticulum calcium release compared in slow-twitch and fast-twitch fibres of mouse muscle. J Physiol 2003; 551(1): 125-38.
[http://dx.doi.org/10.1113/jphysiol.2003.041608] [PMID: 12813151]

[46] Goodman BE. Channels active in the excitability of nerves and skeletal muscles across the neuromuscular junction: basic function and pathophysiology. Adv Physiol Educ 2008; 32(2): 127-35.
[http://dx.doi.org/10.1152/advan.00091.2007] [PMID: 18539851]

[47] Liu W, Olson SD. Compartment calcium model of frog skeletal muscle during activation. J Theor Biol 2015; 364: 139-53.
[http://dx.doi.org/10.1016/j.jtbi.2014.08.050] [PMID: 25234233]

[48] MacIntosh BR. Role of calcium sensitivity modulation in skeletal muscle performance. Physiology (Bethesda) 2003; 18(6): 222-5.

[http://dx.doi.org/10.1152/nips.01456.2003] [PMID: 14614153]

[49] Berridge MJ, Bootman MD, Roderick HL. Calcium signalling: dynamics, homeostasis and remodelling. Nat Rev Mol Cell Biol 2003; 4(7): 517-29.
[http://dx.doi.org/10.1038/nrm1155] [PMID: 12838335]

[50] Eshima H, Tamura Y, Kakehi S, *et al.* Dysfunction of muscle contraction with impaired intracellular Ca^{2+} handling in skeletal muscle and the effect of exercise training in male *db/db* mice. J Appl Physiol 2019; 126(1): 170-82.
[http://dx.doi.org/10.1152/japplphysiol.00048.2018] [PMID: 30433865]

[51] Bruton J, Katz A, Lännergren J, Abbate F, Westerblad H. Regulation of myoplasmic Ca 2+ in genetically obese (ob/ob) mouse single skeletal muscle fibres. Pflugers Arch 2002; 444(6): 692-9.
[http://dx.doi.org/10.1007/s00424-002-0882-1] [PMID: 12355168]

[52] Bayley JS, Pedersen TH, Nielsen OB. Skeletal muscle dysfunction in the db/db mouse model of type 2 diabetes. Muscle Nerve 2016; 54(3): 460-8.
[http://dx.doi.org/10.1002/mus.25064] [PMID: 26833551]

[53] Jaque-Fernandez F, Beaulant A, Berthier C, *et al.* Preserved Ca^{2+} handling and excitation–contraction coupling in muscle fibres from diet-induced obese mice. Diabetologia 2020; 63(11): 2471-81.
[http://dx.doi.org/10.1007/s00125-020-05256-8] [PMID: 32840676]

[54] Muramatsu K, Niwa M, Tamaki T, *et al.* Effect of streptozotocin-induced diabetes on motoneurons and muscle spindles in rats. Neurosci Res 2017; 115: 21-8.
[http://dx.doi.org/10.1016/j.neures.2016.10.004] [PMID: 27826051]

[55] Toth C, Hebert V, Gougeon C, Virtanen H, Mah JK, Pacaud D. Motor unit number estimations are smaller in children with type 1 diabetes mellitus: A case–cohort study. Muscle Nerve 2014; 50(4): 593-8.
[http://dx.doi.org/10.1002/mus.24212] [PMID: 24536037]

[56] Martinez-Pena y Valenzuela I, Akaaboune M. The disassembly of the neuromuscular synapse in high-fat diet-induced obese male mice. Mol Metab 2020; 36: 100979.
[http://dx.doi.org/10.1016/j.molmet.2020.100979] [PMID: 32283080]

[57] Johnson RJ, Segal MS, Sautin Y, *et al.* Potential role of sugar (fructose) in the epidemic of hypertension, obesity and the metabolic syndrome, diabetes, kidney disease, and cardiovascular disease. Am J Clin Nutr 2007; 86(4): 899-906.
[http://dx.doi.org/10.1093/ajcn/86.4.899] [PMID: 17921363]

[58] Jun L, Robinson M, Geetha T, Broderick TL, Babu JR. Prevalence and mechanisms of skeletal muscle atrophy in metabolic conditions. Int J Mol Sci 2023; 24(3): 2973.
[http://dx.doi.org/10.3390/ijms24032973] [PMID: 36769296]

[59] Bellary S, Kyrou I, Brown JE, Bailey CJ. Type 2 diabetes mellitus in older adults: clinical considerations and management. Nat Rev Endocrinol 2021; 17(9): 534-48.
[http://dx.doi.org/10.1038/s41574-021-00512-2] [PMID: 34172940]

[60] Miyake H, Kanazawa I, Tanaka K, Sugimoto T. Low skeletal muscle mass is associated with the risk of all-cause mortality in patients with type 2 diabetes mellitus. Ther Adv Endocrinol Metab 2019; 10: 2042018819842971.
[http://dx.doi.org/10.1177/2042018819842971] [PMID: 31040938]

[61] Ballak SB, Degens H, Busé-Pot T, de Haan A, Jaspers RT. Plantaris muscle weakness in old mice: relative contributions of changes in specific force, muscle mass, myofiber cross-sectional area, and number. Age (Omaha) 2014; 36(6): 9726.
[http://dx.doi.org/10.1007/s11357-014-9726-0] [PMID: 25414077]

CHAPTER 6

The Cellular Mechanism in Skeletal Muscle in Metabolic Disease: Lipid Species and Oxidative Stress

Hiroaki Eshima[1,*]

[1] *Department of International Tourism, Sports Tourism Course, Nagasaki International University, Nagasaki, Japan*

Abstract: Obesity and diabetes impair skeletal muscle metabolism, muscle atrophy, and contractile function, but the intracellular mechanisms have not been clarified fully. Increasing evidence suggests that oxidative stress is associated with obesity and diabetes. Depending on the pathological condition, stress may be affected to a greater extent. Muscle oxidative stress has been implicated in lipid species composition in type 2 diabetes. This chapter discusses the impact of metabolic disease on the regulation of lipid species and oxidative stress.

Keywords: Ferroptosis, Lipid species, Oxidative stress, Phospholipid, Skeletal muscle.

INTRODUCTION

Under obesogenic conditions such as feeding a high-fat diet (HFD), the excessive abundance of fat leads to intramyocellular (IMCL) accumulation [1]. IMCL disrupts muscle function, resulting in muscle atrophy in obese [2, 3] and diabetic mice [4]. These results from IMCL accumulation are associated with increased reactive oxygen species (ROS) production that can compromise the antioxidant defense system of skeletal muscle [5]. However, the specific effect of lipid species on oxidative stress in skeletal muscle has not been clarified fully.

Oxidative stress is important for skeletal muscle atrophy [6]. For example, long-term inactivity, such as tail suspension, immobilization, and small cage housing, promote oxidative stress and result in muscle atrophy [7 - 9]. This inactivity-induced muscle atrophy increases intracellular ROS production. Recent studies have indicated that redox signaling is an important regulator of cell signaling pat-

---

[*] **Corresponding author Hiroaki Eshima:** Department of International Tourism, Sports Tourism Course, Nagasaki International University, Nagasaki, Japan; E-mail: heshima@niu.ac.jp

Hiroaki Eshima, Ikuru Miura, Yutaka Matsunaga & Yuki Tomiga (Eds.)

hways [10]. Similar to these findings, increased ROS production is an important signal for muscle atrophy induced by aging [11] and cancer [12]. Recent evidence indicates obesity and diabetes induce ROS production [13 - 15], suggesting that metabolic imbalance is linked to dysfunction of the cellular redox system.

The excess lipids are susceptible to oxidation induced by free radicals. Lipid hydroperoxides (LOOH) are one of the primary products of lipid hydroperoxidation and induce oxidative stress. Recently, Stockwell identified that ferroptosis is a novel cell death mechanism characterized by iron-dependent lipid peroxidation [16]. Ferroptosis is associated with a variety of diseases, including cancer, kidney diseases, atherosclerosis, and liver diseases, suggesting that ferroptosis can provide insights and treatment strategies for metabolic diseases [17].

In this chapter, we will discuss the evidence that oxidative stress, particularly lipid peroxidation, contributes to the cell signaling pathways for skeletal muscle homeostasis.

LIPID SPECIES IN SKELETAL MUSCLE

Lipids act as structural components of cell membranes and energy storage sources and participate in signaling pathways. They are also ubiquitous in the organism and play diverse biochemical and physiological functions. Lipid species are present in many classes and can transduce signals to influence cell function (Table 1).

Table 1. Categories of lipid molecular species.

Category	Specific Lipid Species
Fatty acyls	Fatty acids, elcosanoids, endocannabinoids
Glycerolipids	TAG, diacylglycerols
Glycerophospholipid	PC, PE, PI, PS, PG, PA, CL
Sphingolipids	Sphingomyelin, sulfatides, sphingosine, ceramides, ganglioside
Sterol lipids	Cholesterol, estradiol, testosterone, bile acids
Prenol lipids	Farnesol, dolichols, vitamin K
Saccharolipids	Lipid A, acyltrehaloses
Polyketides	Aflatoxins, tetracyclines, erythromycin

In metabolic disease, obese and type 2 diabetes mellitus (T2DM) patients increase concentration of plasma free fatty acid (FFA) [18]. An increased FFA was observed in skeletal muscles from obese rodents [19 - 21] and in obese and T2DM patients [22, 23]. Plasma FFA enters intramyocellular lipids*via* protein transporters, such as fatty acid translocase, fatty acid binding protein, and fatty acid transport protein family [24]. Then, fatty acids attach coenzyme A in a reaction catalyzed by acyl-Co synthase and formatted of long-chain acyl-CoA. These are used as a substrate in *de novo* synthesis of other lipids, including triacylglycerols (TAG), diacylglycerols (DAG), and ceramides [25, 26].

In skeletal muscle, a previous study demonstrates that lipid extracts using mass spectrometry analysis have the presence of lipid species, including phospholipids, sphingolipids, and cholesterol esters [27]. The main fatty acid is TAG, and most extracellular-derived fatty acids enter the pool of intracellular TAG [28, 29]. Obesity generally changes lipid species content, including fatty acids of phospholipid and triglyceride [30, 31] (Figs. **1**-**3**). Particularly, obese muscle exhibits increased polyunsaturated (PUFA) from phospholipid and triglyceride fractions [31]. Indeed, analyzing fatty acid-related metabolism, many genes are significantly changed in obese muscle. Consistent with this, obesity increases the fatty acid of phospholipid molecular species.

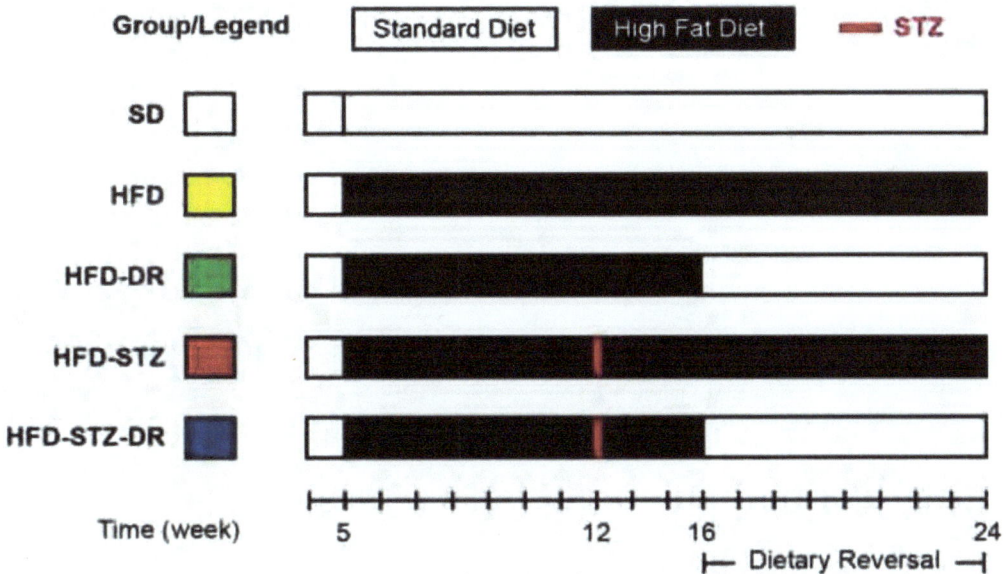

Fig. (1). Experimental design from a previous study. Animals began HFD at 5 and 12 weeks; two cohorts were administered STZ to induce a T2D phenotype. At 16 weeks, a cohort of HFD and HFD-STZ mice were placed on the standard diet (SD) for 8 weeks. From [32].

In humans, triglyceride and phospholipid content in skeletal muscle have been linked to insulin sensitivity [33 - 35]. Indeed, skeletal muscle phospholipids are inversely related to body fat [35] (Fig. **4**). Skeletal muscles are also influenced by environmental factors such as diet and exercise. Endurance training causes alteration of fatty acid composition and triglycerides in skeletal muscle [36]. Taken together, lipid species may regulate muscle metabolism, but the underlying mechanisms are not completely understood.

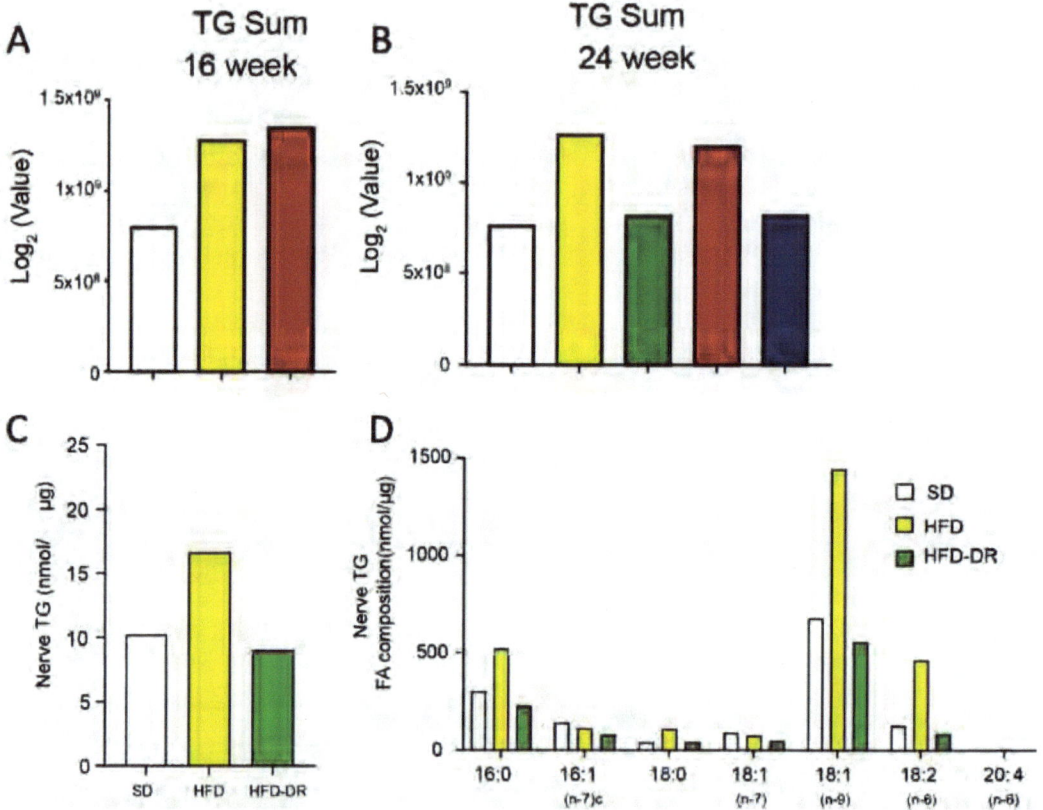

Fig. (2). The triglyceride content of nerve from obese (**A**) and T2DM (**B**) models. Increased TG from obesity is reversible by weight loss-induced standard diet feeding (**C** and **D**). From [32].

NOVEL POTENTIAL MECHANISMS FOR OXIDATIVE STRESS IN METABOLIC DISEASE

Oxidative stress is activated in the early stages of oxidation and can be regulated by various factors. Intracellular reactive oxygen species (ROS) are often generated by mitochondrial oxidative phosphorylation and formed as intermediates of oxidoreductase enzymes. Oxygen atoms are susceptible to radical formation because they contain two unpaired electrons in separate orbits of their outer electron shell. ROS including superoxide anion (O_2^-), hydrogen peroxide (H_2O_2), hydroxyl radical ($^\cdot OH$), hypochlorous acid (HOCl), peroxynitrite anion ($ONOO^-$), and nitric oxide (N_O). They are radical or non-radical molecules that can react with a wide spectrum of molecules and change their structures in a reversible manner [37, 38] (Fig. **5**).

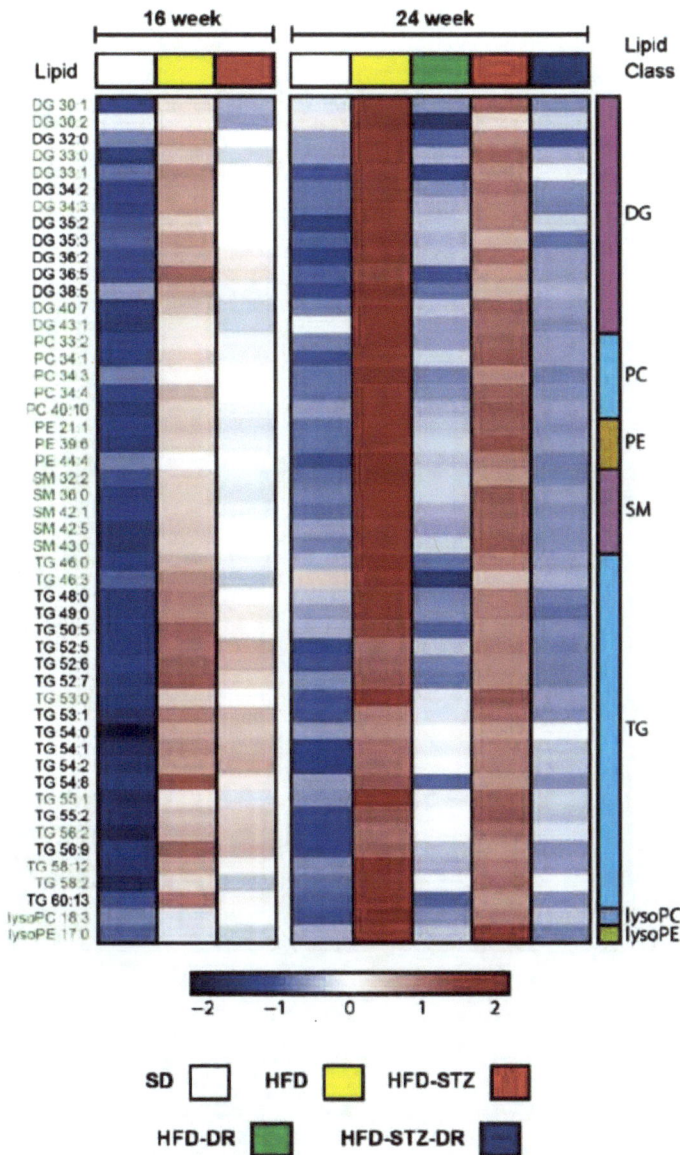

Fig. (3). Obesity and type 2 diabetes generally change lipid species content, including fatty acids of phospholipid and triglyceride. From [32].

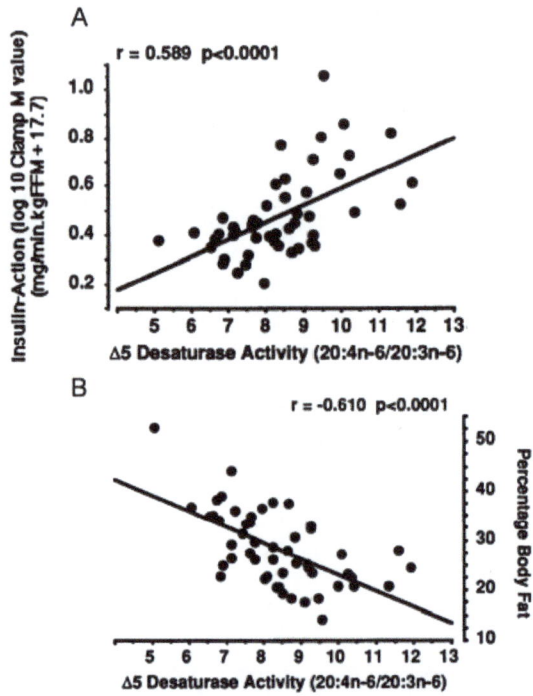

Fig. (4). Relationship between muscle phospholipid and insulin sensitivity (**A**) and percentage of body fat (**B**). From [35].

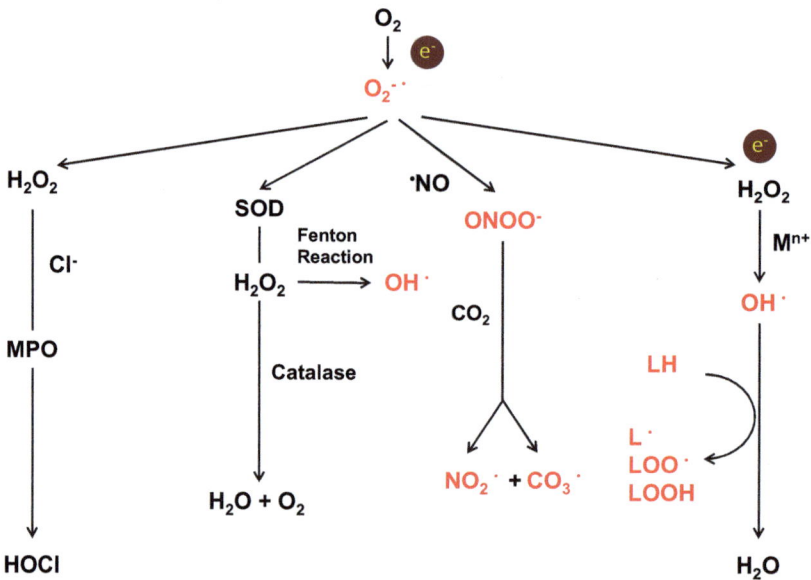

Fig. (5). Reduction of oxygen and its byproducts. H_2O_2: Hydrogen Peroxide; MPO: myeloperoxidase; HOCl: Hypochlorous acid; SOD: superoxide dismutase; OH•: Hydroxyl radical; NO: nitric oxide; ONOO: peroxynitrite; LH: lipid; LOO •: peroxidized lipid radical; LOOH: peroxide lipid: LH; L•: lipid radical.

H_2O_2 is a byproduct of reactive oxygen that serves as a main regulator for oxidative stress. In skeletal muscle, H_2O_2 produced by NADPH oxidase 2 (NOX2) is involved in insulin action [39, 40]. The •OH is a main cellular redox state, and its dysregulation impacts various pathologies. The •OH is highly reactive with other molecules to achieve stability. The •OH is a harmful byproduct of oxidative metabolism, which can cause cell damage. It shows an average lifetime of 10-9 nanoseconds and can react with nearly every biomolecule.

ROS have been implicated in muscle atrophy caused by a variety of disease states, including aging [41], physical inactivity [6], and cachexia [42], as well as metabolic diseases, including obesity and diabetes, which cause muscle wasting together with accumulation of ROS [43]. However, the mechanisms of oxidative stress in muscle atrophy have not been completely elucidated. Because ROS refers to a collection of radical molecules whose cellular signals are vast, it is unclear which ROS molecules are responsible for the loss of muscle mass and function that occurs with disease. ROS signaling includes those that are essential for health; it is important to identify the downstream effector of ROS that promotes metabolic insult.

Accumulation of ROS will affect organelles and cell membranes and lead to alteration of gene expression and proteins through apoptosis, calcium flux, and proteolysis. Oxidative stress is the production of superoxide anions by the mitochondrial electron transport chain (ETC). The impairment of mitochondrial biogenesis by obesity has been implicated in both reactive lipid accumulation and increased ROS production [44 - 46], but some data present are negative data from rodent and human studies [47, 48]. Therefore, the mechanism of mitochondrial ROS for the skeletal muscle of metabolic disorders has not been clarified fully.

Lipid hydroperoxides are oxidized cellular phospholipids that have the ability to self-propagate and cause oxidative stress [49]. Lipid hydroperoxides were initially discovered to induce a form of non-apoptotic iron-dependent cell death coined ferroptosis in 2012 [16]. Since then, lipid hydroperoxides have been identified to play a role in a variety of diseases, including motor neuron degeneration [50], cardiovascular [51], tumor [52], and obesity [14]. Notably, recent studies elucidated the role of lipid hydroperoxides in sarcopenia [53, 54]. Aging decreases the expression of Gpx4 in skeletal muscle (Fig. **6**). Aging also increases over 300 species of oxidized lipids. It has a robust effect on oxidized PE, lipids implicated as a potential lipid signal to induce ferroptosis [55] (Fig. **7**). Lipid hydroperoxides may be suppressed and rendered nonreactive *via* glutathione peroxidase 4 (Gpx4), which acts to neutralize lipid hydroperoxides to nonreactive lipid alcohol [56]. Interestingly, Gpx4-overexpressing transgenic mice could be protected from disuse-induced skeletal muscle atrophy and weakness [54].

Furthermore, pharmacologic suppression of lipid carbonyl stress by N-acetylcarnosine treatment also prevented decreases in muscle mass and force-generating induced by age and disuse. As shown in Fig. (**2**), these studies suggest that lipid hydroperoxides are an important downstream contributor of ROS to promote sarcopenia [54].

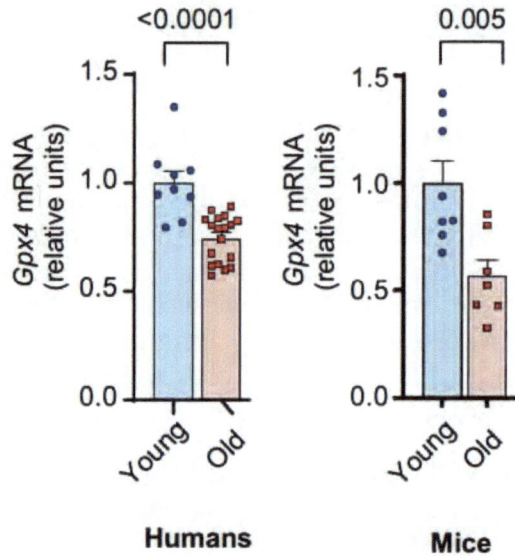

Fig. (6). Glutathione peroxidase 4 (Gpx4) mRNA levels in skeletal muscle biopsy samples from young and old humans or gastrocnemius muscles from young and old mice. From [54].

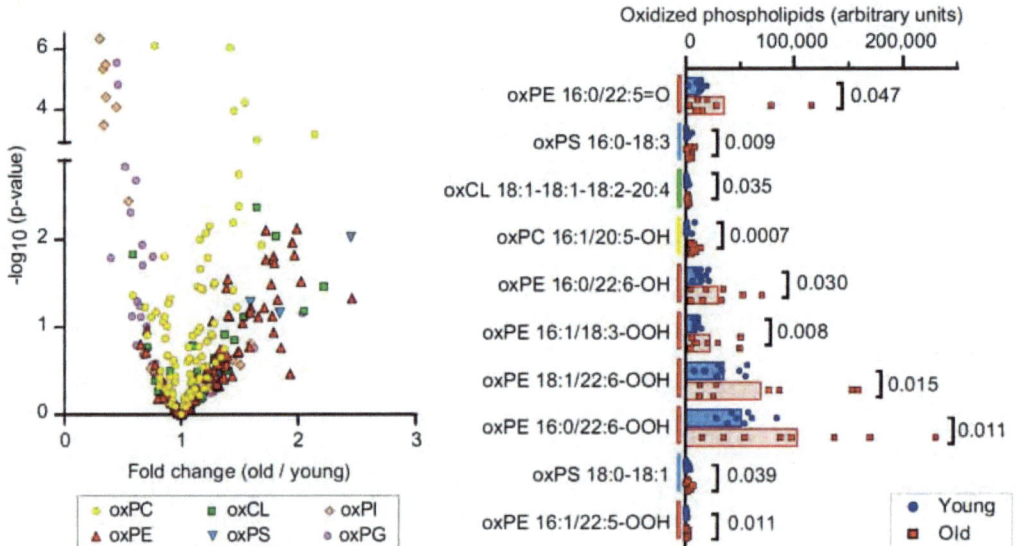

Fig. (7). Oxidized phospholipid content in gastrocnemius muscles from young and old male mice. From [54].

Lipid hydroperoxides have long been linked with worsened metabolic health in metabolic disease [57]. Metabolic insult may cause increased lipid content in circulation, which is easily attacked by ROS and gives rise to lipid peroxidation. Indeed, lipid peroxidation significantly increased in patients with T2DM, and there is a significant positive correlation between lipid aldehyde levels and HbA1c [58].

Ferroptosis inducers identified Erastin, an inhibitor of cystine import *via* system X_c^- which subsequently causes depletion of glutathione and covalent inhibitors of Gpx4 [59]. In contrast, Ferrostatin-1, a potent and selective ferroptosis inhibitor, prevents lipid peroxidation in cancer cells [60]. Ferroptosis inhibitors also have already been investigated in the management of diabetes [61]. Several studies demonstrated the association of ferroptosis with inflammation, beta-cell death, insulin resistance, and diabetes models [62 - 64]. However, the role of lipid peroxidation on metabolic insult-induced muscle atrophy is not fully understood, and further investigations are required to clarify the mechanisms (Fig. **8**).

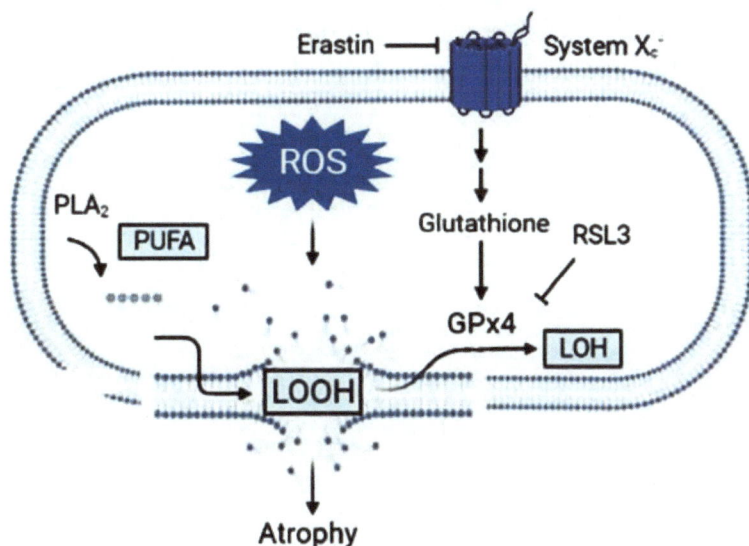

Fig. (8). A schematic diagram of muscle atrophy associated with lipid hydroperoxide.

Exercise and shivering are two examples of an increase in whole-body energy expenditure through energy expenditure in muscles. Exercise improves obesity and glucose homeostasis in patients with type 2 diabetes [65]. Indeed, the acceleration of glucose uptake into skeletal muscle by endurance exercise training is well-established [66]. Shivering thermogenic mechanisms may partially affect whole-body metabolism and weight gain. Cold acclimation has been shown to alter skeletal muscle metabolism and mostly improve whole-body energy expenditure. A previous study shows that cold acclimation increased insulin sensitivity and muscle GLUT4 translocation in type 2 diabetes subjects, suggesting that cold exposure may be a potential therapy for diabetes [67]. On the other hand, cold exposure causes ferroptosis in multiple cell lines [68]. Indeed, chronic cold stress induces oxidative stress injury through the ferroptosis pathway in the liver and pancreas from Yorkshire pig models [69]. Consistent with pig models, oxidative damage accumulates in muscles as a response to cold stress in rodent models [70]. Currently, the mechanism underlying cold stress and ferroptosis has not been fully elucidated, and further investigations are required to clarify the mechanisms.

CONCLUDING REMARKS

This chapter discusses the impact of metabolic disorders on morphology and function in skeletal muscle. The potential mechanism of loss of muscle mass and contractile dysfunction in metabolic disorders has not been fully clarified. If future studies allow us to determine potential cellular mechanisms, they may provide clues for therapeutic strategies to promote skeletal muscle health and improve the overall quality of life.

REFERENCES

[1]   Unger RH, Clark GO, Scherer PE, Orci L. Lipid homeostasis, lipotoxicity and the metabolic syndrome. Biochim Biophys Acta Mol Cell Biol Lipids 2010; 1801(3): 209-14.
        [http://dx.doi.org/10.1016/j.bbalip.2009.10.006] [PMID: 19948243]

[2]   Poggiogalle E, Lubrano C, Gnessi L, *et al.* The decline in muscle strength and muscle quality in relation to metabolic derangements in adult women with obesity. Clin Nutr 2019; 38(5): 2430-5.
        [http://dx.doi.org/10.1016/j.clnu.2019.01.028] [PMID: 30792144]

[3]   Sousa LGO, Marshall AG, Norman JE, *et al.* The effects of diet composition and chronic obesity on muscle growth and function. J Appl Physiol 2021; 130(1): 124-38.
        [http://dx.doi.org/10.1152/japplphysiol.00156.2020] [PMID: 33211595]

[4]   Yamamoto H, Eshima H, Kakehi S, Kawamori R, Watada H, Tamura Y. Impaired fatigue resistance, sarcoplasmic reticulum function, and mitochondrial activity in soleus muscle of db/db mice. Physiol Rep 2022; 10(18): e15478.
        [http://dx.doi.org/10.14814/phy2.15478] [PMID: 36117307]

[5]   Rains JL, Jain SK. Oxidative stress, insulin signaling, and diabetes. Free Radic Biol Med 2011; 50(5): 567-75.
        [http://dx.doi.org/10.1016/j.freeradbiomed.2010.12.006] [PMID: 21163346]

[6]   Powers SK, Smuder AJ, Criswell DS. Mechanistic links between oxidative stress and disuse muscle atrophy. Antioxid Redox Signal 2011; 15(9): 2519-28.
        [http://dx.doi.org/10.1089/ars.2011.3973] [PMID: 21457104]

[7]   Powers SK, Smuder AJ, Judge AR. Oxidative stress and disuse muscle atrophy. Curr Opin Clin Nutr Metab Care 2012; 15(3): 240-5.
        [http://dx.doi.org/10.1097/MCO.0b013e328352b4c2] [PMID: 22466926]

[8]   Yoshihara T, Natsume T, Tsuzuki T, *et al.* Long-term physical inactivity exacerbates hindlimb unloading-induced muscle atrophy in young rat soleus muscle. J Appl Physiol 2021; 130(4): 1214-25.
[http://dx.doi.org/10.1152/japplphysiol.00494.2020] [PMID: 33600278]

[9]   Nuoc TN, Kim S, Ahn SH, Lee JS, Park BJ, Lee TH. The analysis of antioxidant expression during muscle atrophy induced by hindlimb suspension in mice. J Physiol Sci 2017; 67(1): 121-9.
[http://dx.doi.org/10.1007/s12576-016-0444-5] [PMID: 26971264]

[10] Powers SK, Schrager M. Redox signaling regulates skeletal muscle remodeling in response to exercise and prolonged inactivity. Redox Biol 2022; 54: 102374.
[http://dx.doi.org/10.1016/j.redox.2022.102374] [PMID: 35738088]

[11] Foreman NA, Hesse AS, Ji LL. Redox signaling and sarcopenia: searching for the primary suspect. Int J Mol Sci 2021; 22(16): 9045.
[http://dx.doi.org/10.3390/ijms22169045] [PMID: 34445751]

[12] Huot JR, Baumfalk D, Resendiz A, Bonetto A, Smuder AJ, Penna F. Targeting mitochondria and oxidative stress in cancer- and chemotherapy-induced muscle wasting. Antioxid Redox Signal 2023; 38(4-6): 352-70.
[PMID: 36310444]

[13] Nelson MAM, Efird JT, Kew KA, *et al.* Enhanced catecholamine flux and impaired carbonyl metabolism disrupt cardiac mitochondrial oxidative phosphorylation in diabetes patients. Antioxid Redox Signal 2021; 35(4): 235-51.
[http://dx.doi.org/10.1089/ars.2020.8122] [PMID: 33066717]

[14] Anderson EJ, Vistoli G, Katunga LA, *et al.* A carnosine analog mitigates metabolic disorders of obesity by reducing carbonyl stress. J Clin Invest 2018; 128(12): 5280-93.
[http://dx.doi.org/10.1172/JCI94307] [PMID: 30226473]

[15] Anderson EJ, Lustig ME, Boyle KE, *et al.* Mitochondrial H_2O_2 emission and cellular redox state link excess fat intake to insulin resistance in both rodents and humans. J Clin Invest 2009; 119(3): 573-81.
[http://dx.doi.org/10.1172/JCI37048] [PMID: 19188683]

[16] Dixon SJ, Lemberg KM, Lamprecht MR, *et al.* Ferroptosis: an iron-dependent form of nonapoptotic cell death. Cell 2012; 149(5): 1060-72.
[http://dx.doi.org/10.1016/j.cell.2012.03.042] [PMID: 22632970]

[17] Lee JY, Kim WK, Bae KH, Lee SC, Lee EW. Lipid metabolism and ferroptosis. Biology (Basel) 2021; 10(3): 184.
[http://dx.doi.org/10.3390/biology10030184] [PMID: 33801564]

[18] Belfort R, Mandarino L, Kashyap S, *et al.* Dose-response effect of elevated plasma free fatty acid on insulin signaling. Diabetes 2005; 54(6): 1640-8.
[http://dx.doi.org/10.2337/diabetes.54.6.1640] [PMID: 15919784]

[19] Blachnio-Zabielska AU, Chacinska M, Vendelbo MH, Zabielski P. The crucial role of C18-Cer in fat-induced skeletal muscle insulin resistance. Cell Physiol Biochem 2016; 40(5): 1207-20.
[http://dx.doi.org/10.1159/000453174] [PMID: 27960149]

[20] Blachnio-Zabielska AU, Razak Hady H, Markowski AR, *et al.* Inhibition of ceramide *de novo* synthesis affects adipocytokine secretion and improves systemic and adipose tissue insulin sensitivity. Int J Mol Sci 2018; 19(12): 3995.
[http://dx.doi.org/10.3390/ijms19123995] [PMID: 30545025]

[21] Grycel S, Markowski AR, Hady HR, *et al.* Metformin treatment affects adipocytokine secretion and lipid composition in adipose tissues of diet-induced insulin-resistant rats. Nutrition 2019; 63-64: 126-33.
[http://dx.doi.org/10.1016/j.nut.2019.01.019] [PMID: 30959381]

[22] Roepstorff C, Wulff Helge J, Vistisen B, Kiens B. Studies of plasma membrane fatty acid-binding protein and other lipid-binding proteins in human skeletal muscle. Proc Nutr Soc 2004; 63(2): 239-44.

[http://dx.doi.org/10.1079/PNS2004332] [PMID: 15294037]

[23] Bruce CR, Anderson MJ, Carey AL, *et al.* Muscle oxidative capacity is a better predictor of insulin sensitivity than lipid status. J Clin Endocrinol Metab 2003; 88(11): 5444-51.
[http://dx.doi.org/10.1210/jc.2003-030791] [PMID: 14602787]

[24] Schwieterman W, Sorrentino D, Potter BJ, *et al.* Uptake of oleate by isolated rat adipocytes is mediated by a 40-kDa plasma membrane fatty acid binding protein closely related to that in liver and gut. Proc Natl Acad Sci USA 1988; 85(2): 359-63.
[http://dx.doi.org/10.1073/pnas.85.2.359] [PMID: 3277174]

[25] Grevengoed TJ, Klett EL, Coleman RA. Acyl-CoA metabolism and partitioning. Annu Rev Nutr 2014; 34(1): 1-30.
[http://dx.doi.org/10.1146/annurev-nutr-071813-105541] [PMID: 24819326]

[26] Turner N, Cooney GJ, Kraegen EW, Bruce CR. Fatty acid metabolism, energy expenditure and insulin resistance in muscle. J Endocrinol 2014; 220(2): T61-79.
[http://dx.doi.org/10.1530/JOE-13-0397] [PMID: 24323910]

[27] Borg ML, Andrews ZB, Duh EJ, Zechner R, Meikle PJ, Watt MJ. Pigment epithelium-derived factor regulates lipid metabolism *via* adipose triglyceride lipase. Diabetes 2011; 60(5): 1458-66.
[http://dx.doi.org/10.2337/db10-0845] [PMID: 21464445]

[28] Bessesen DH, Rupp CL, Eckel RH. Trafficking of dietary fat in lean rats. Obes Res 1995; 3(2): 191-203.
[http://dx.doi.org/10.1002/j.1550-8528.1995.tb00135.x] [PMID: 7719965]

[29] Dyck DJ, Bonen A. Muscle contraction increases palmitate esterification and oxidation and triacylglycerol oxidation. Am J Physiol 1998; 275(5): E888-96.
[PMID: 9815010]

[30] Werner JU, Tödter K, Xu P, *et al.* Comparison of fatty acid and gene profiles in skeletal muscle in normal and obese C57BL/6J mice before and after blunt muscle injury. Front Physiol 2018; 9: 19.
[http://dx.doi.org/10.3389/fphys.2018.00019] [PMID: 29441023]

[31] Montgomery MK, Brown SHJ, Mitchell TW, Coster ACF, Cooney GJ, Turner N. Association of muscle lipidomic profile with high-fat diet-induced insulin resistance across five mouse strains. Sci Rep 2017; 7(1): 13914.
[http://dx.doi.org/10.1038/s41598-017-14214-1] [PMID: 29066734]

[32] O'Brien PD, Guo K, Eid SA, *et al.* Integrated lipidomic and transcriptomic analyses identify altered nerve triglycerides in mouse models of prediabetes and type 2 diabetes. Dis Model Mech 2020; 13(2): dmm042101.
[http://dx.doi.org/10.1242/dmm.042101] [PMID: 31822493]

[33] Borkman M, Storlien LH, Pan DA, Jenkins AB, Chisholm DJ, Campbell LV. The relation between insulin sensitivity and the fatty-acid composition of skeletal-muscle phospholipids. N Engl J Med 1993; 328(4): 238-44.
[http://dx.doi.org/10.1056/NEJM199301283280404] [PMID: 8418404]

[34] Clore JN, Li J, Gill R, *et al.* Skeletal muscle phosphatidylcholine fatty acids and insulin sensitivity in normal humans. Am J Physiol 1998; 275(4): E665-70.
[PMID: 9755086]

[35] Pan DA, Lillioja S, Milner MR, *et al.* Skeletal muscle membrane lipid composition is related to adiposity and insulin action. J Clin Invest 1995; 96(6): 2802-8.
[http://dx.doi.org/10.1172/JCI118350] [PMID: 8675650]

[36] Andersson A, Sjödin A, Hedman A, Olsson R, Vessby B. Fatty acid profile of skeletal muscle phospholipids in trained and untrained young men. Am J Physiol Endocrinol Metab 2000; 279(4): E744-51.
[http://dx.doi.org/10.1152/ajpendo.2000.279.4.E744] [PMID: 11001754]

[37]   Liochev SI. Reactive oxygen species and the free radical theory of aging. Free Radic Biol Med 2013; 60: 1-4.
[http://dx.doi.org/10.1016/j.freeradbiomed.2013.02.011] [PMID: 23434764]

[38]   Bouviere J, Fortunato RS, Dupuy C, Werneck-de-Castro JP, Carvalho DP, Louzada RA. Exercise-stimulated ros sensitive signaling pathways in skeletal muscle. Antioxidants 2021; 10(4): 537.
[http://dx.doi.org/10.3390/antiox10040537] [PMID: 33808211]

[39]   Espinosa A, Campos C, Díaz-Vegas A, *et al.* Insulin-dependent H_2O_2 production is higher in muscle fibers of mice fed with a high-fat diet. Int J Mol Sci 2013; 14(8): 15740-54.
[http://dx.doi.org/10.3390/ijms140815740] [PMID: 23899788]

[40]   Dohm GL, Tapscott EB, Pories WJ, *et al.* An *in vitro* human muscle preparation suitable for metabolic studies. Decreased insulin stimulation of glucose transport in muscle from morbidly obese and diabetic subjects. J Clin Invest 1988; 82(2): 486-94.
[http://dx.doi.org/10.1172/JCI113622] [PMID: 3403714]

[41]   Scicchitano BM, Pelosi L, Sica G, Musarò A. The physiopathologic role of oxidative stress in skeletal muscle. Mech Ageing Dev 2018; 170: 37-44.
[http://dx.doi.org/10.1016/j.mad.2017.08.009] [PMID: 28851603]

[42]   Ábrigo J, Elorza AA, Riedel CA, *et al.* Role of oxidative stress as key regulator of muscle wasting during cachexia. Oxid Med Cell Longev 2018; 2018(1): 2063179.
[http://dx.doi.org/10.1155/2018/2063179] [PMID: 29785242]

[43]   D'Souza DM, Al-Sajee D, Hawke TJ. Diabetic myopathy: impact of diabetes mellitus on skeletal muscle progenitor cells. Front Physiol 2013; 4: 379.
[http://dx.doi.org/10.3389/fphys.2013.00379] [PMID: 24391596]

[44]   Bonnard C, Durand A, Peyrol S, *et al.* Mitochondrial dysfunction results from oxidative stress in the skeletal muscle of diet-induced insulin-resistant mice. J Clin Invest 2008; 118(2): 789-800.
[http://dx.doi.org/10.1172/JCI32601] [PMID: 18188455]

[45]   Lefort N, Glancy B, Bowen B, *et al.* Increased reactive oxygen species production and lower abundance of complex I subunits and carnitine palmitoyltransferase 1B protein despite normal mitochondrial respiration in insulin-resistant human skeletal muscle. Diabetes 2010; 59(10): 2444-52.
[http://dx.doi.org/10.2337/db10-0174] [PMID: 20682693]

[46]   Matsunami T, Sato Y, Sato T, Ariga S, Shimomura T, Yukawa M. Oxidative stress and gene expression of antioxidant enzymes in the streptozotocin-induced diabetic rats under hyperbaric oxygen exposure. Int J Clin Exp Pathol 2009; 3(2): 177-88.
[PMID: 20126586]

[47]   Abdul-Ghani MA, Jani R, Chavez A, Molina-Carrion M, Tripathy D, DeFronzo RA. Mitochondrial reactive oxygen species generation in obese non-diabetic and type 2 diabetic participants. Diabetologia 2009; 52(4): 574-82.
[http://dx.doi.org/10.1007/s00125-009-1264-4] [PMID: 19183935]

[48]   Paglialunga S, van Bree B, Bosma M, *et al.* Targeting of mitochondrial reactive oxygen species production does not avert lipid-induced insulin resistance in muscle tissue from mice. Diabetologia 2012; 55(10): 2759-68.
[http://dx.doi.org/10.1007/s00125-012-2626-x] [PMID: 22782287]

[49]   Miranda ER, Shahtout JL, Funai K. Chicken or egg? mitochondrial phospholipids and oxidative stress in disuse-induced skeletal muscle atrophy. Antioxid Redox Signal 2023; 38(4-6): 338-51.
[PMID: 36301935]

[50]   Chen L, Hambright WS, Na R, Ran Q. Ablation of the ferroptosis inhibitor glutathione peroxidase 4 in neurons results in rapid motor neuron degeneration and paralysis. J Biol Chem 2015; 290(47): 28097-106.
[http://dx.doi.org/10.1074/jbc.M115.680090] [PMID: 26400084]

[51]   Miró O, Casademont J, Casals E, *et al.* Aging is associated with increased lipid peroxidation in human hearts, but not with mitochondrial respiratory chain enzyme defects. Cardiovasc Res 2000; 47(3): 624-31.
[http://dx.doi.org/10.1016/S0008-6363(00)00122-X] [PMID: 10963736]

[52]   Jiang L, Kon N, Li T, *et al.* Ferroptosis as a p53-mediated activity during tumour suppression. Nature 2015; 520(7545): 57-62.
[http://dx.doi.org/10.1038/nature14344] [PMID: 25799988]

[53]   Czyżowska A, Brown J, Xu H, *et al.* Elevated phospholipid hydroperoxide glutathione peroxidase (GPX4) expression modulates oxylipin formation and inhibits age-related skeletal muscle atrophy and weakness. Redox Biol 2023; 64: 102761.
[http://dx.doi.org/10.1016/j.redox.2023.102761] [PMID: 37279604]

[54]   Eshima H, Shahtout JL, Siripoksup P, *et al.* Lipid hydroperoxides promote sarcopenia through carbonyl stress. eLife 2023; 12: e85289.
[http://dx.doi.org/10.7554/eLife.85289] [PMID: 36951533]

[55]   Kagan VE, Mao G, Qu F, *et al.* Oxidized arachidonic and adrenic PEs navigate cells to ferroptosis. Nat Chem Biol 2017; 13(1): 81-90.
[http://dx.doi.org/10.1038/nchembio.2238] [PMID: 27842066]

[56]   Yang WS, SriRamaratnam R, Welsch ME, *et al.* Regulation of ferroptotic cancer cell death by GPX4. Cell 2014; 156(1-2): 317-31.
[http://dx.doi.org/10.1016/j.cell.2013.12.010] [PMID: 24439385]

[57]   Shabalala SC, Johnson R, Basson AK, *et al.* Detrimental effects of lipid peroxidation in type 2 diabetes: exploring the neutralizing influence of antioxidants. Antioxidants 2022; 11(10): 2071.
[http://dx.doi.org/10.3390/antiox11102071] [PMID: 36290794]

[58]   Fatani SH, Babakr AT, NourEldin EM, Almarzouki AA. Lipid peroxidation is associated with poor control of type-2 diabetes mellitus. Diabetes Metab Syndr 2016; 10(2) (Suppl. 1): S64-7.
[http://dx.doi.org/10.1016/j.dsx.2016.01.028] [PMID: 26806326]

[59]   Xie Y, Hou W, Song X, *et al.* Ferroptosis: process and function. Cell Death Differ 2016; 23(3): 369-79.
[http://dx.doi.org/10.1038/cdd.2015.158] [PMID: 26794443]

[60]   Skouta R, Dixon SJ, Wang J, *et al.* Ferrostatins inhibit oxidative lipid damage and cell death in diverse disease models. J Am Chem Soc 2014; 136(12): 4551-6.
[http://dx.doi.org/10.1021/ja411006a] [PMID: 24592866]

[61]   Prasad M K, Mohandas S, Kunka Mohanram R. Role of ferroptosis inhibitors in the management of diabetes. Biofactors 2023; 49(2): 270-96.
[http://dx.doi.org/10.1002/biof.1920] [PMID: 36468443]

[62]   Miao R, Fang X, Zhang Y, Wei J, Zhang Y, Tian J. Iron metabolism and ferroptosis in type 2 diabetes mellitus and complications: mechanisms and therapeutic opportunities. Cell Death Dis 2023; 14(3): 186.
[http://dx.doi.org/10.1038/s41419-023-05708-0] [PMID: 36882414]

[63]   Yang XD, Yang YY. Ferroptosis as a novel therapeutic target for diabetes and its complications. Front Endocrinol (Lausanne) 2022; 13: 853822.
[http://dx.doi.org/10.3389/fendo.2022.853822] [PMID: 35422764]

[64]   Li S, Li Y, Wu Z, Wu Z, Fang H. Diabetic ferroptosis plays an important role in triggering on inflammation in diabetic wound. Am J Physiol Endocrinol Metab 2021; 321(4): E509-20.
[http://dx.doi.org/10.1152/ajpendo.00042.2021] [PMID: 34423682]

[65]   Sylow L, Kleinert M, Richter EA, Jensen TE. Exercise-stimulated glucose uptake — regulation and implications for glycaemic control. Nat Rev Endocrinol 2017; 13(3): 133-48.
[http://dx.doi.org/10.1038/nrendo.2016.162] [PMID: 27739515]

[66]   Frøsig C, Rose AJ, Treebak JT, Kiens B, Richter EA, Wojtaszewski JFP. Effects of endurance exercise training on insulin signaling in human skeletal muscle: interactions at the level of phosphatidylinositol 3-kinase, Akt, and AS160. Diabetes 2007; 56(8): 2093-102.
[http://dx.doi.org/10.2337/db06-1698] [PMID: 17513702]

[67]   Hanssen MJW, Hoeks J, Brans B, *et al.* Short-term cold acclimation improves insulin sensitivity in patients with type 2 diabetes mellitus. Nat Med 2015; 21(8): 863-5.
[http://dx.doi.org/10.1038/nm.3891] [PMID: 26147760]

[68]   Hattori K, Ishikawa H, Sakauchi C, Takayanagi S, Naguro I, Ichijo H. Cold stress-induced ferroptosis involves the ASK 1-p38 pathway. EMBO Rep 2017; 18(11): 2067-78.
[http://dx.doi.org/10.15252/embr.201744228] [PMID: 28887319]

[69]   Teng T, Zheng Y, Zhang M, *et al.* Chronic cold stress promotes inflammation and ER stress *via* inhibiting GLP-1R signaling, and exacerbates the risk of ferroptosis in the liver and pancreas. Environ Pollut 2024; 360: 124647.
[http://dx.doi.org/10.1016/j.envpol.2024.124647] [PMID: 39089475]

[70]   Venditti P, Di Stefano L, Di Meo S. Vitamin E reduces cold-induced oxidative stress in rat skeletal muscle decreasing mitochondrial H_2O_2 release and tissue susceptibility to oxidants. Redox Rep 2009; 14(4): 167-75.
[http://dx.doi.org/10.1179/135100009X466113] [PMID: 19695124]

SUBJECT INDEX

www.ingramcontent.com/pod-product-compliance
Lightning Source LLC
Chambersburg PA
CBHW041720210326
41598CB00007B/723